Recent Results in Cancer Research

153

Managing Editors
P. M. Schlag, Berlin · H.-J. Senn, St. Gallen

Associate Editors
V. Diehl, Cologne · D.M. Parkin, Lyon
M.F. Rajewsky, Essen · R. Rubens, London
M. Wannenmacher, Heidelberg

Founding Editor
P. Rentchnik, Geneva

Springer

Berlin
Heidelberg
New York
Barcelona
Hong Kong
London
Milan
Paris
Singapore
Tokyo

K. Höffken   R. Kath   (Eds.)

Peptides in Oncology III

Somatostatin and LH-RH Analogues

With 14 Figures and 14 Tables

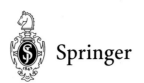

Springer

Prof. Dr. med. Klaus Höffken
Priv.-Doz. Dr. med. Roland Kath
Klinik und Poliklinik für Innere Medizin,
Innere Medizin II (Hämatologie, Onkologie,
Endokrinologie, Stoffwechselerkrankungen)
Klinikum der Friedrich-Schiller-Universität Jena
Erlanger Allee 101
D-07740 Jena

ISBN 3-540-64429-6 Springer-Verlag Berlin Heidelberg New York
ISSN 0080-0015

1 80183 4212

Library of Congress Cataloging-in-Publication Data

Peptides in oncology: somatostatin and LH-RH analogues / K. Hoffken, R. Kath, eds. p. cm.
– (Recent results in cancer research, ISSN 0080-0015; 153) Includes bibliographical references and index. ISBN 3-540-64429-6 (hardcover: alk. paper). 1. Luteinizing hormone
releasing hormone – Derivatives – Therapeutic use. 2. Somatostatin – Derivatives – Therapeutic use. 3. Cancer – Hormone therapy. I. Hoffken, K. (Klaus), 1946 –. II. Kath, R.
(Roland), 1957 –. III. Series [DNLM: 1. Neoplasms – drug therapy. 2. Somatostatin –
therapeutic use. 3. Somatostatin – analogs & derivatives. 4. Gonadorelin – therapeutic
use. 5. Gonadorelin – analogs & derivatives. W1RE106P. v. 153 1998]. RC261.R35 vol. 153
[RC271.L87] 616.99′4061 – dc21 DNLM/DLC for Library of Congress.

Production: PRO EDIT GmbH, D-69126 Heidelberg
Typesetting: K+V Fotosatz GmbH, D-64743 Beerfelden

SPIN 10671510   21/3133-5 4 3 2 1 0 – Printed on acid-free paper

Preface

Interference with protein-mediated intra- and intercellular pathways has become a major goal of preclinical and clinical research. A rapidly increasing number of peptides are known to be responsible for endo-, para- and autocrine signal transduction. These peptides and their receptors have been studied with regard to their cell growth stimulatory action and their impact on differentiation. In parallel, peptide antagonists are being investigated in terms of their potential role in preclinical and clinical application. Thus, biotherapy might improve the clinical outcome of patients with tumors that respond to the respective hormonal manipulation.

Among the numerous peptides of interest somatostatin (somatotropin release inhibitory factor) and the luteinizing hormone releasing hormone (LH-RH) have been the topic of intensive research during recent years. In this third volume of peptides in oncology, experts in the field extensively review and update the mechanisms of action of somatostatin and LH-RH-analogues in oncology.

Somatostatin and its various short- and long-acting analogues have the unique feature of suppressing and inhibiting a wide range of cellular processes including cell proliferation. Receptors for these peptides which belong to the family of neuropeptides or neurotransmitters, are widely distributed, a feature which is not in keeping with the general view of a growth hormone regulatory system. LH-RH analogues play an established role in curative (adjuvant) and palliative treatment of hormone sensitive tumors. Furthermore, the effect of LH-RH analogues is mediated through specific receptors assuring principally an antiproliferative effect even in estrogen receptor-negative tumors.

Krenning and coworkers report on their experiences of end-stage patients with mainly neuroendocrine tumors administering radioactive somatostatin. The theoretical background of new molecular aspects in the diagnosis and therapy of neuroendocrine gastroentero-pancreatic tumors is throughly illustrated by Pape and coworkers. Furthermore, the role of somatostatin and its analgoues in the endocrine gastroentero-pancreatic tumors as well as other carcinomas is reviewed in two chapters by Fehlmann et al. and Kath and Höffken. Finally, the classical hormone responsive tumors (breast, ovarian and prostate cancer) are discussed. Preclinical and clinical findings regarding established and new LH-RH analgoues are demonstrated by Höffken and Kath, Altwein and Emmons and coworkers.

We trust that this volume on peptides in oncology will update the knowledge of these substances in tumor diagnosis and antineoplastic therapy. It is our belief that the search for the best peptide analogues, perhaps in combination with other treatment strategies, will result in improvement of clinical outcome for tumor patients.

Jena, Autumn 1999   R. Kath
                                                               K. Höffken

Contents

List of Contributors *

Altwein, J. E.[71]
Arnold, R.[15]
Bakker, W. H.[1]
Breeman, W. A. P.[1]
de Herder, W. W.[1]
de Jong, M.[1]
Emons, G.[83]
Fehmann, H.-C.[15]
Höcker, M.[45]
Höffken, K.[23, 61]
Jamar, F.[1]
Kath, R.[23, 61]

Kooij, P. P. M.[1]
Krenning, E. P.[1]
Kwekkeboom, D. J.[1]
Pape, U.-F.[45]
Pauwels, S.[1]
Schulz, K.-D.[83]
Seuß, U.[45]
Valkema, R.[1]
van Eijck, C. H. J.[1]
Wiedenmann, B.[45]
Wulbrand, U.[15]

---

* The address of the principal author is given on the first page of each contribution.
[1] Page on which contribution begins.

The Role of Radioactive Somatostatin and Its Analogues in the Control of Tumor Growth

E. P. Krenning[1,2], R. Valkema[1], P. P. M. Kooij[1], W. A. P. Breeman[1],
W. H. Bakker[1], W. W. de Herder[2], C. H. J. van Eijck[3],
D. J. Kwekkeboom[1], M. de Jong[1], F. Jamar[4], and S. Pauwels[4]

[1] University Hospital and Erasmus University Rotterdam (EUR), Department of Nuclear Medicine, Dr. Molewaterplein 40, 3015 GD Rotterdam, The Netherlands
[2] Department of Internal Medicine III, University Hospital and Erasmus University Rotterdam (EUR), The Netherlands
[3] Department of Surgery, University Hospital and Erasmus University Rotterdam (EUR), The Netherlands
[4] Department of Nuclear Medicine, Catholic University of Louvain, Brussels, Belgium

Abstract

Peptide receptor scintigraphy with the radioactive somatostatin analogue [^{111}In-DTPA-D-Phe^1]octreotide is a sensitive and specific technique to show in vivo the presence and abundance of somatostatin receptors on various tumors. With this technique primary tumors and metastases of neuroendocrine cancers as well as of many other cancer types can be localized. This technique is currently used to assess the possibility of peptide receptor radionuclide therapy with repeated administration of high doses of [^{111}In-DTPA-D-Phe^1]octreotide. ^{111}In emits Auger and conversion electrons, having a tissue penetration of 0.02–10 µm and 200–500 µm, respectively. Thirty end-stage patients with mostly neuroendocrine progressing tumors were treated with [^{111}In-DTPA-D-Phe^1]octreotide, up to a maximal cumulative patient dose of about 74 GBq, in a phase-I trial. There were no major clinical side effects after up to 2 years of treatment, except that in a few patients a transient decline in platelet counts and lymphocyte subsets occurred. Promising beneficial effects on clinical symptoms, hormone production, and tumor proliferation were found. Of the 21 patients who received a cumulative dose of more than 20 GBq, eight showed stabilization of disease and six others a reduction in tumor size. There is a tendency towards better results in patients whose tumors have a higher accumulation of the radioligand. Peptide receptor radionuclide therapy is also feasible with ^{111}In as the radionuclide. Theoretically, depending on the homogeneity of distribution of tumor cells expressing peptide receptors and the size of the tumor, β-emitting radionuclides, e.g., ^{90}Y, labeled to DOTA-chelated peptides may

Recent Results in Cancer Research, Vol. 153
© Springer-Verlag Berlin · Heidelberg 2000

be more effective than ^{111}In for peptide receptor radionuclide therapy. The first peptide receptor radionuclide therapy trials with [90Y-DOTA-Tyr3]octreotide started recently.

Introduction

Peptide receptor scintigraphy with the radioactive somatostatin analogue, [111In-DTPA-D-Phe1]octreotide, is a sensitive and specific technique to show in vivo the presence and abundance of somatostatin receptors on various tumors. In general, mapping of the presence of various peptide receptors on the cell membrane by peptide receptor scintigraphy (PRS) may become an attractive, noninvasive, harmless, easy-to-use tool for an individual therapeutic approach to the cancer patient (Breeman et al. 1996; Krenning et al. 1993, 1995; Virgolini et al. 1994). The detection of heterogeneous metastases (with regard to the expression of different peptide receptors or the accumulation of other radiolabeled ligands) also becomes possible if a combination of radiolabeled peptides or of radiolabeled peptides with other radioligands (all labeled with different radionuclides) can be used. At the moment, examples of this approach are the use of (a) octreotide and MIBG scintigraphy in patients with metastasized pheochromocytomas and (b) octreotide and radioiodine scintigraphy in patients with metastasized differentiated thyroid cancer. One of the therapeutic options for patients with endocrine cancers is the use of nonradioactive peptides (or antagonists), but the use of radiolabeled peptides, possibly in combination with other radiolabeled ligands (e.g., MIBG or radioiodine) may become a new alternative or adjunct therapy.

Several radionuclides for coupling to [DTPA-D-Phe1]octreotide have been proposed and investigated in radiotherapeutic applications (Fig. 1). [90]Y, a suitable β-emitting radionuclide, shows dissociation from this chelated peptide in serum. ^{111}In-labeled [DTPA-D-Phe1]octreotide has an appropriate distribution profile in human beings for PRS and peptide receptor radionuclide therapy (PRRT; Krenning et al. 1994, 1996). [111]In emits Auger and conversion electrons and can therefore be used to investigate what antiproliferative effect it may have in cancer.

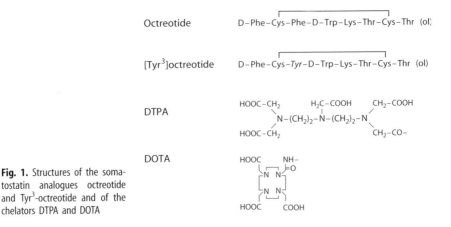

Fig. 1. Structures of the somatostatin analogues octreotide and Tyr³-octreotide and of the chelators DTPA and DOTA

Scintigraphy with [¹¹¹In-DTPA-D-Phe¹]octreotide

The efficacy of PRS with [¹¹¹In-DTPA-D-Phe¹]octreotide (somatostatin receptor scintigraphy) was evaluated in a European multicenter trial (EMT) of 350 patients with a histologically or biochemically proven gastroenteropancreatic (GEP) tumor (Krenning et al. 1995). Tumor sites were detected by conventional imaging methods (CIM) in 88%, whereas somatostatin receptor scintigraphy was positive in 80%. The highest success rates of somatostatin receptor scintigraphy were observed with glucagonomas (100%), vipomas (88%), carcinoids (87%), and nonfunctioning islet cell tumors (ICT) (82%). The low detection rate (46%) noted for insulinomas is related to the lower incidence of subtype 2 (sst2) somatostatin receptors on insulinoma cells. However, the overall 80% sensitivity found is somewhat lower than the 88% obtained at Erasmus University Rotterdam (EUR) in 130 patients with GEP tumors. This may be related to important differences in scanning procedures, such as the amount of radioligand administered (minimal dose of ¹¹¹In of 200 MBq and at least 10 µg of peptide at EUR), the duration of the acquisition, and the use of single photon emission computed tomography (SPECT) (with a triple-head camera at EUR). The fact that abdominal SPECT was not systematically performed in all patients of the EMT may explain why only 73% of gastrinoma patients had a positive scan compared with the 90–100% sensitivity reported in other studies. In the EMT, a total of 388 sites were visualized with CIM in 308 of the 350 patients. In addition to 297 known localizations, somatostatin receptor scintigraphy revealed another 166 unsuspected lesions. Forty percent of these unsuspected lesions were subsequently confirmed as true-positive findings based on the results of additional imaging procedures or histology obtained during the 1-year follow-up period. The clinical relevance of detecting additional tumor localizations is very dependent on the clinical status of the patient. The demonstration of an unsuspected lesion in a patient with known metastatic spread usually has little impact on the management. In contrast, the detection of unsuspected tumor sites in patients with a single known lesion or without any known lesion is important, in that it may affect the selection for curative surgery, which remains the treatment of choice for patients with this type of tumor. In the cohort of 350 patients studied, 42 had no lesion detected by CIM and 178 were known to have a single tumor localization prior to the study. Somatostatin receptor scintigraphy was positive in 11 of the 42 patients (25%), and 12 of 16 lesions revealed by somatostatin receptor scintigraphy were further confirmed as true positive. Somatostatin receptor scintigraphy demonstrated multiple tumor sites in 62 of the 178 patients (35%); 60% of these lesions were confirmed by follow-up (1 year) procedures. A reply to an impact questionnaire was obtained from 235 patients; overall, the scintigraphic findings led to management changes in 40%.

In a prospective study Gibril et al. (1996) compared the sensitivity of somatostatin receptor scintigraphy with that of CT, MRI, ultrasonography, and selective angiography in the detection of primary and metastatic gastrinomas. They concluded that somatostatin receptor scintigraphy is the single most sensitive method for imaging either primary or metastatic liver lesions in patients with Zollinger-Ellison syndrome. The same group studied the effect of somatostatin receptor scintigraphy on clinical management based on the data of this comparative study (Gibril et al. 1996; Termanini et al. 1997). Since this technique altered management for 47% of the patients, they concluded that somatostatin receptor scintigraphy should be the initial imaging modality for patients with gastrinomas, also because of its superior sensitivity, high specificity, simplicity, and cost-effectiveness. Furthermore, it is likely that the conclusion drawn from this study can also be extended to other pancreatic endocrine tumor syndromes with the exception of insulinomas (Termanini et al. 1997).

Radionuclide Therapy with [^{111}In-DTPA-D-Phe^1]octreotide

The side effects and antiproliferative effect of multiple high radiotherapeutic doses of [^{111}In-DTPA-D-Phe^1]octreotide, using the Auger and conversion electrons emitted by ^{111}In, are being investigated in patients and are reported here preliminarily (Fjalling et al. 1996; Krenning et al. 1994, 1996). In this phase-1 study of therapy with [^{111}In-DTPA-D-Phe^1]octreotide we included mainly end-stage patients with a high tumor load of progressing neuroendocrine tumors.

Materials and Methods

[DTPA-D-Phe^1]octreotide (Fig. 1) and ^{111}InCl$_3$ (DRN 4901, 370 MBq/ml in HCl, pH 1.5–1.9) were obtained from Mallinckrodt Medical BV (Petten, The Netherlands). [DTPA-D-Phe1]octreotide was labeled with ^{111}In as described previously (Bakker et al. 1991). Since 1995, the typical doses per administration are 6000–7000 MBq ^{111}In incorporated in 40–50 µg [DTPA-D-Phe^1]octreotide within 24 h after production of ^{111}In. It is given with at least 2-week intervals between administrations, and a total of eight administrations is aimed at with extensions to 12–14 administrations. Radionuclide therapy with [^{111}In-DTPA-D-Phe^1]octreotide was applied after we had received witnessed informed consent by the patient and approval by the medical ethics committee of our hospital.

The following measurements, carried out prior to and between all administrations, served as parameters of possible side effects: the usual hematological and chemical analyses of bone marrow, liver, kidney, and endocrine pancreatic (glucose or Hb A$_{1c}$) function. Pituitary function (free T4; postmenopausal women: LH and FSH; men: testosterone) was assessed prior to and 4 weeks after the fourth and eighth administration of [111In-DTPA-D-Phe^1]octreotide: at these time points also possible effects on (a) the endocrine activity of the tumors and/or their production of specific serum markers, and (b) tumor size (CT or MRI) were investigated. Pituitary-adrenal-axis function (metyrapone test) prior to and after eight administrations as well as at long-term follow-up with 3- to 4-month intervals was also investigated, if feasible.

Scoring of tumor radioactivity uptake prior to the start of treatment with [^{111}In-DTPA-D-Phe^1]octreotide was done visually using scintigrams obtained 24 h after injection of a diagnostic dose (220 MBq) of [^{111}In-DTPA-D-Phe^1]octreotide. The scoring grades used were 4 = intense, 3 = clear (higher than liver uptake), 2 = clear but faint (lower than or equal to liver uptake), 1 = equivocal, and 0 = no accumulation.

Patients were also scanned 3 and 7 days after each administration of the radiotherapeutic dose. Percentage uptake of the administered dose in total body and in the most prominent tumor were calculated (data not shown). Uptake decreased slowly or remained the same if the interval between the successive administrations was less than 1 month. In patients who received six or more administrations of 6000–7000 MBq [^{111}In-DTPA-D-Phe^1]octreotide at maximal intervals of 1 month, uptake in the tumor was still clearly visible after the last administration. Typical radiation doses to tissues with administered doses of 6000–7000 MBq [^{111}In-DTPA-D-Phe1]octreotide are: kidneys 300–1400 cGy [depending on the relative biological effectiveness (RBE, 1–20) for Auger electrons], spleen 200 cGy, liver 50 cGy, bone marrow 13 cGy (target organ for gamma photons), thyroid gland 25 cGy, and pituitary 70 cGy (Krenning et al. 1992). Thus the critical organs are kidneys and spleen. With these administered doses the estimated tumor radiation doses for a 10-g tumor are (assumptions: 1% uptake; effective half-life is equal to the physical half-life) 1700 and 6700 cGy (RBE for Auger electrons 1 and 20, respectively) and for a 100-g tumor (1% uptake) 250 and 750 cGy, respectively.

Results and Discussion

Thirty end-stage patients with mainly neuroendocrine tumors have been treated with [^{111}In-DTPA-D-Phe^1]octreotide in Rotterdam ($n = 29$) and Brussels ($n = 1$) (Table 1). Twenty-one of these 30 patients received a total cumulative dose of at least 20 GBq [^{111}In-DTPA-D-Phe^1]octreotide. Of the nine patients treated with a total dose lower than 20 GBq, seven had to stop prematurely because of progressive disease despite the treatment with [^{111}In-DTPA-D-Phe^1]octreotide and two have not yet concluded the first of four courses. The tumor uptake scores in the seven patients with very progressive disease varied between 2 ($n = 3$), 3 ($n = 2$), and 4 ($n = 2$).

Multiple high radiotherapeutic doses of [^{111}In-DTPA-D-Phe^1]octreotide were given to 21 patients up to total cumulative doses of 22–30 GBq and to 12 patients up to 50–60 GBq per patient. Three patients received maximum doses of about 75 GBq [^{111}In-DTPA-D-Phe^1]octreotide. No major side effects were noticed in the first treated patient after a cumulative dose of 25 GBq and a follow-up interval of

Table 1. Characteristics of patients treated with [^{111}In-DTPA-D-Phe[1]]octreotide (*P* progression, *S* stable, *R* reduction in tumor size)

	n	Grade II	Grade III	Grade IV
Carcinoid	10	1 (P)	6 (2[a], P, 2 S, R)	3 (2[a], S)
NE tumor	7	1 (R)	3 (2[a], P)	3 (P, S, R)
Gastrinoma	1		1 (S)	
Vipoma	1			1 (R)
Glucagonoma	1			1 (R)
Med. thyroid cancer	4	4 (1[a], 2 P, S)		
Pap. thyroid cancer	2	2 (1[a], S)		
Glomus tumor	1			1 (R)
Pheochromocytoma	2	2 (P, S)		
Leiomyosarcoma	1	1 (1[a])		
Total	21 (+9[a])	8 (+3[a])	6 (+4[a])	7 (+2[a])
Positive effect (S+R)	67%	50%	67%	86%

[a] $\ll$20 GBq and/or no FU.

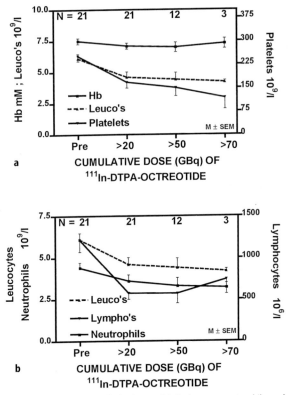

Fig. 2 a, b. Course of blood cells (**a** hemoglobin, leukocytes, and platelets and **b** leukocytes, neutrophils, and lymphocytes) during peptide receptor radionuclide treatment with the indicated cumulative doses of [^{111}In-DTPA-D-Phe[1]]octreotide. *n* = number of patients

2 years, the longest follow-up period so far. In the other patients no major clinical side effects were observed either.

Figure 2 shows the course of blood cells and platelet counts. Radiotherapy with [^{111}In-DTPA-D-Phe^1]octreotide may (transiently) affect the number of white blood cells and, to an even greater extent, that of platelets.

Renal function was monitored by measurements of serum creatinine and creatinine clearance (Fig. 3). If there is any effect on the kidney function it is of no clinical relevance so far. It is remarkable that the average kidney function of the seven patients with creatinine clearances between 21 and 80 ml/min prior to the start of PRRT did not significantly change after administrations of cumulative doses of 20–30 GBq ($n=7$) and 50–60 GBq ($n=3$) with a maximum follow-up of 2 years.

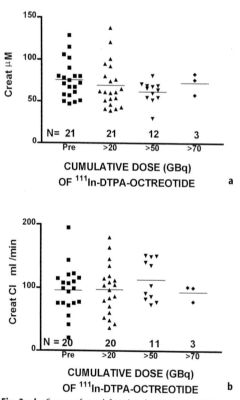

Fig. 3 a, b. Course of renal function (**a** serum creatinine and **b** creatinine clearance) during peptide receptor radionuclide treatment with the indicated cumulative doses of [^{111}In-DTPA-D-Phe^1]octreotide. n=number of patients

It is well known that the pituitary and pancreatic islet cells express somatostatin receptors. Endocrine parameters of pituitary and pancreatic function during treatment cycles and follow-up after treatment with [^{111}In-DTPA-D-Phe^1]octreotide did not change either (data not shown).

Impressive, though in a number of patients temporary because of end-stage disease, effects on the clinical condition of the patient and on hormone or tumor marker production (overall data not shown; Fig. 4) were observed following administration of multiple high doses of [^{111}In-DTPA-D-Phe^1]octreotide. Also, anti-proliferative effects have been noticed (Fig. 5). All 21 patients who received a total cumulative dose of at least 20 GBq ^{111}In-labeled [DTPA-D-Phe^1]octreotide had progressive disease, i.e., unequivocal increase in tumor volume according to CT or MRI prior to the start of [^{111}In-DTPA-D-Phe^1]octreotide therapy. In eight patients this treatment resulted in stable disease and in another six patients in actual tumor shrinkage. Thus, six of 21 patients with progressive disease who received an adequate dose of at least 20 GBq [^{111}In-DTPA-D-Phe^1]octreotide showed an antiproliferative effect. So far, it may be concluded that a response to treatment with [^{111}In-DTPA-D-Phe^1]octreotide, based on antiproliferative effects and a lowering of tumor markers in serum and/or urine, was obtained when (a) the cumulative therapeutic dose of

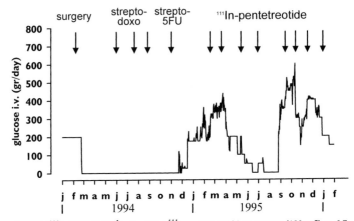

Fig. 4. The endocrine effect of [^{111}In-DTPA-D-Phe^1]octreotide (*^{111}In-pentetreotide*) treatment (180-mCi or 6.7-GBq doses) in a patient with a very progressive, metastasized neuroendocrine tumor of the pancreas producing, among other hormones, insulin, leading to profound hypoglycemia, which forced permanent hospitalization for i.v. glucose administration. Between the fourth and fifth administration of [^{111}In-DTPA-D-Phe^1]octreotide the patient was discharged for a short period, during which no special precautions had to be taken to maintain euglycemia. Some tumors showed regression and others an increase in size. The effect of PRRT in this patient has been scored in the table as "progression." The patient died in February 1996

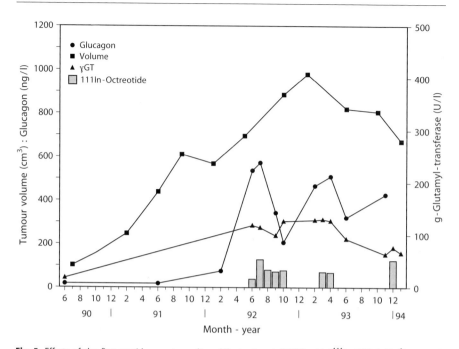

Fig. 5. Effects of the first peptide receptor radionuclide treatment (PRRT) with [^{111}In-DTPA-D-Phe^1]octreotide in a patient with metastasized glucagonoma. Other treatment modalities, e.g., surgery, high doses of octreotide without and with interferon-α, were ineffective prior to the start of PRRT in August 1992. *Tumor volume* is total abdominal tumor load based on measurements of all lesions shown on CT. Note that the decline in tumor size starts at a time point at which the total abdominal tumor load is about 1 kg. The total reduction in tumor size was 35%. The treatment protocol in this case is different from the present one described under Material and Methods. The experience with the first two patients (second patient with glomus tumor) formed the basis of our present treatment protocol

[^{111}In-DTPA-D-Phe^1]octreotide was at least about 20 GBq and (b) tumor uptake was at least grade 2 in order to get a stabilization of disease and grade 3 or 4 for reduction in size of tumors (Table 1).

The observed responses to this peptide receptor radionuclide therapy are in agreement with internalization of [^{111}In-DTPA-D-Phe^1]octreotide into tumor cells [because of the abundance of Auger and conversion electrons with a (very) short particle range or tissue penetration] and with an antiproliferative effect induced by these electrons. Since at present it is not exactly known to what extent and where the radionuclide is localized intracellularly after administration of high amounts of [^{111}In-DTPA-D-Phe^1]octreotide, measurements of the actual radiation doses are not possible. However, one of the possible intracellular locations is the lysosomal compartment (Andersson et al. 1996; Duncan et al. 1997).

It is to be expected that the radiotherapeutic use of radionuclides such as ^{90}Y, emitting the higher energies of β-particles and coupled to (small) DOTA-chelated peptides, leads to higher radiation doses in a larger part of the tumor, also because of their more appropriate particle ranges or tissue penetration (de Jong et al. 1997; Otte et al. 1997). In contrast to [^{90}Y-DTPA-D-Phe[1]]octreotide, ^{90}Y-labeled [DOTA-Tyr[3]]octreotide shows no dissociation from this DOTA-chelated peptide in serum. The first two peptide receptor radionuclide therapy trials with [^{90}Y-DOTA-Tyr[3]]octreotide started recently (Otte et al. 1998; Krenning, Kvols, Pauwels in Novartis B151 trial). Based on the assumptions stated in the preceding section and on a similar biodistribution (^{111}In-and ^{90}Y-labeled peptide), the estimated tumor radiation dose after an administered dose of 3.7 GBq ^{90}Y-labeled peptide will be 16 500 cGy (10 g, 1% uptake) and 1800 cGy (100 g, 1% uptake). Estimated tissue doses are 2400 cGy for the kidneys (without co-infusion of amino acids), 150 cGy for the liver, and 1400 cGy for the spleen. Thus, tumors with an inhomogeneous distribution of cells expressing peptide receptors may respond more favorably to this kind of treatment because of the better cross fire. Of course, one might also anticipate more side effects with PRRT when ^{90}Y is used. For instance, the better tissue penetration of ^{90}Y localized in tubular cells may affect the glomeruli and eventually induce a glomerular fibrosis. Measures have to be taken to decrease the renal accumulation of β-emitting peptides when they are used for PRRT, e.g., with lysine infusions and NH_4Cl (Bernard et al. 1997; de Jong et al. 1996). In this study, in which [^{111}In-DTPA-D-Phe[1]]octreotide was used, no special precautions were taken to lower renal uptake.

In this phase-1 study of therapy with [^{111}In-DTPA-D-Phe[1]]octreotide we included only end-stage patients with (neuroendocrine) tumors expressing a (rather) homogeneous distribution of somatostatin receptors and preferably high or modest accumulation of the radioligand. Based on our results with [^{111}In-DTPA-D-Phe[1]]octreotide scintigraphy and given a relatively high accumulation of the radioligand in the tumor, it is anticipated that patients with the following tumors might be candidates for this kind of treatment: most (metastasized) GEP tumors and paragangliomas and 30% and 40% of malignant lymphomas and small cell lung cancers, respectively.

References

Andersson P, Forssel-Aronsson E, Johanson V, Wangberg B, Nilsson O, Fjalling M, Ahlman H (1996) Internalization of indium-111 into human neuroendocrine tumor cells after incubation with indium-111-DTPA-D-Phe1-octreotide. J Nucl Med 37:2002–2006

Bakker WH, Albert R, Bruns C, Breeman WAP, Hofland LJ, Marbach P, Pless J, Pralet D, Stolz B, Koper JW, Lamberts SWJ, Visser TJ, Krenning EP (1991) [111In-DTPA-D-Phe1]-octreotide, a potential radiopharmaceutical for imaging of somatostatin receptor-positive tumors: synthesis, radiolabeling and in vitro validation. Life Sci 49:1583–1591

Bernard HF, Krenning EP, Breeman WAP, Rolleman EJ, Bakker WH, Visser TJ, Macke H, de Jong M (1997) D-lysine reduction of indium-111 octreotide and yttrium-90 octreotide renal uptake. J Nucl Med 38:1929–1934

Breeman WA, van Hagen MP, Visser-Wisselaar HA, van der Pluijm ME, Koper JW, Setyono-Han B, Bakker WH, Kwekkeboom DJ, Hazenberg MP, Lamberts SW, Visser TJ, Krenning EP (1996) In vitro and in vivo studies of substance P receptor expression in rats with the new analog [indium-111-DTPA-Arg1] substance P. J Nucl Med 37:108–117

de Jong M, Rolleman EJ, Bernard BF, Visser TJ, Bakker WH, Breeman WAP, Krenning EP (1996) Inhibition of renal uptake of indium-111-DTPA-octreotide in vivo. J Nucl Med 37:1388–1392

de Jong M, Bakker WH, Krenning EP, Breeman WAP, van der Pluijm ME, Bernard BF, Visser TJ, Jermann E, Behe M, Powell P, Macke HR (1997) Yttrium-90 and indium-111 labelling, receptor binding and biodistribution of [DOTA0, D-Phe1, Tyr3]octreotide, a promising somatostatin analogue for radionuclide therapy. Eur J Nucl Med 24:368–371

Duncan JR, Stephenson MT, Wu HP, Anderson CJ (1997) Indium-111-diethylene-triamine-pentaacetic acid-octreotide is delivered in vivo to pancreatic, tumor cell, renal, and hepatocyte lysosomes. Cancer Res 57:659–671

Fjalling M, Andersson P, Forssell-Aronsson E, Gretarsdottir J, Johansson V, Tisell LE, Wangberg B, Nilsson O, Berg G, Michanek A, Lindstedt G, Ahlman H (1996) Systemic radionuclide therapy using indium-111-DTPA-D-Phe1-octreotide in midgut carcinoid syndrome. J Nucl Med 37:1519–1521

Gibril F, Reynolds JC, Doppman JL, Chen CC, Venzon DJ, Termanini B, Weber HC, Stewart CA, Jensen RT (1996) Somatostatin receptor scintigraphy: its sensitivity compared with that of other imaging methods in detecting primary and metastatic gastrinomas. Ann Intern Med 125:26–34

Krenning EP, Bakker WH, Kooij PPM, Breeman WAP, Oei HY, de Jong M, Reubi JC, Visser TJ, Bruns C, Kwekkeboom DJ, Reijs AEM, van Hagen PM, Koper JW, Lamberts SWJ (1992) Somatostatin receptor scintigraphy with [111In DTPA-D-Phe1]octreotide in man: metabolism, dosimetry and comparison with [123I-Tyr3]octreotide. J Nucl Med 33:652–658

Krenning EP, Kwekkeboom DJ, Bakker WH, Breeman WAP, Kooij PPM, Oei HY, van Hagen M, Postema PTE, de Jong M, Reubi JC, Visser TJ, Reijs AEM, Hofland LJ, Koper JW, Lamberts SWJ (1993) Somatostatin receptor scintigraphy with [111In-DTPA-D-Phe1]-and [123I-Tyr3]-octreotide: the Rotterdam experience with more than 1000 patients. Eur J Nucl Med 20:716–731

Krenning EP, Kooij PPM, Bakker WH, Breeman WAP, Postema PTE, Kwekkeboom DJ, Oei HY, de Jong M, Visser TJ, Reijs AEM, Lamberts SWJ (1994) Radiotherapy with a radiolabeled somatostatin analogue, [111In-DTPA-D-Phe1]-octreotide. A case history. Ann NY Acad Sci 733:496–506

Krenning EP, Kwekkeboom DJ, Pauwels S, Kvols LK, Reubi J-C (1995) Somatostatin receptor scintigraphy. In: Freeman LM (ed) Nuclear medicine annual. Raven, New York, pp 1–50

Krenning EP, Kooij PPM, Pauwels S, Breeman WAP, Postema PTE, de Herder WW, Valkema R, Kwekkeboom DJ (1996) Somatostatin receptor: scintigraphy and radionuclide therapy. Digestion 57 [Suppl]:57–61

Otte A, Jermann E, Behe M, Goetze M, Bucher HC, Roser HW, Heppeler A, Mueller-Brand J, Maecke H.(1997) Dotatoc: a powerful new tool for receptor-mediated radionuclide therapy. Eur J Nucl Med 24:792–795

Otte A, Mueller-Brand J, Dellas S, Nitzsche EU, Hermann R, Maecke HR (1998) Yttrium-90-labelled somatostatin analogue for cancer treatment. Lancet 351:417–418

Termanini B, Gibril F, Reynolds JC, Doppman JL, Chen CC, Stewart CA, Sutliff VE, Jensen RT (1997) Value of somatostatin receptor scintigraphy: a prospective study in gastrinoma of its effect on clinical management. Gastroenterology 112:335–347

Virgolini I, Raderer M, Kurtaran, Angelberger P, Banyai S, Yang Q, Li S, Banyai M, Pidlich J, Niederle B, Scheithauer W, Valent P (1994) Vasoactive intestinal peptide receptor imaging for the localization of intestinal adenocarcinomas and endocrine tumors. N Engl J Med 331:1116–1121

Treatment of Endocrine Gastroenteropancreatic Tumors with Somatostatin Analogues

H.-C. Fehmann, U. Wulbrand, and R. Arnold

Division of Gastroenterology and Endocrinology, Department of Medicine, Philipps-University of Marburg, Baldingerstrasse, 35033 Marburg, Germany

Abstract

Somatostatin is a hormone that regulates the function of several exocrine and endocrine glands. The peptide mediates its actions via five different receptors. These proteins are expressed in a tissue-specific manner. Somatostatin receptors are also present in neuroendocrine gastroenteropancreatic tumors. Two long-acting somatostatin analogues, octreotide and lanreotide, are recognized by the receptor subtypes 2 and 5. Excessive hormone secretion in carcinoid syndrome can be controlled by these drugs. In addition, at least a subgroup of patients with carcinoid syndromes respond with delayed tumor growth during octreotide therapy. In the future, the availability of the somatostatin receptor cDNAs will allow the development of specific and even more potent receptor analogues.

Introduction

Somatostatin was originally isolated from the hypothalamus as a tetradecapeptide and described as a growth hormone release inhibitor (Brazeau et al. 1973). Subsequent studies demonstrated that different forms of somatostatin are synthesized in a variety of organs. The most important somatostatin forms consist of 14 and 28 amino acids. They are encoded by a single mRNA, and the common precursor is the subject of tissue-specific post-translational processing (Montminy et al. 1984). Depending upon its target tissue, somatostatin acts as a neurotransmitter, regulates exocrine and endocrine glands, gastrointestinal motility, and vasotone, or influences cell growth and proliferation and immunological processes. In this context it is important to mention that peptides (cortistatins) with a high degree of sequence homology to somatostatin have recently been isolated (de Lecea et al. 1996; Fukusumi et al. 1997). Their physiological role is still not very well defined. The most

Recent Results in Cancer Research, Vol. 153
© Springer-Verlag Berlin · Heidelberg 2000

important intracellular effectors of somatostatin include adenylate cyclase, phospholipase C, ion channels, tyrosine phosphatases, and Na^+/H^+ exchangers. All biological actions of somatostatin are mediated via specific receptors. Actually, five different somatostatin receptor subtypes (SSTR) have been isolated and characterized.

Both somatostatin-14 and -28 have very short biological half-lives in vivo. Therefore, stable analogues for clinical use have been developed. Two of them, octreotide and lanreotide, are actually used on a regular basis (Lamberts et al. 1996). They are stable much longer than the naturally occurring peptides and their therapeutic application is accompanied by only minor side effects, if any. The naturally occurring targets for somatostatin as well as its analogues are the endogenously expressed somatostatin receptors.

Somatostatin Receptors

From 1992 to 1997, five different cDNAs encoding for somatostatin receptors were isolated. They were named sstr 1–5, according to their chronological discovery. Each sstr is the product of a single gene located on a different chromosome (for review see Fehmann and Arnold 1996). Structurally, the sstr belong to the superfamily of G-protein coupled receptors characterized by seven transmembrane domains. The extracellular part is responsible for ligand binding, while the intracellular domains transduce the signal into the cell. Amino acid sequence comparisons show intra- and interspecies homologies of between 35 and 99%.

All five receptors bind somatostatin-14 with the same affinity, while somatostatin-28 is preferably recognized by sstr 5. From a therapeutic point of view, sstr 2 and sstr 5 are the most important receptor subtypes since the clinically used somatostatin analogues octreotide and lanreotide are recognized by these receptors.

sstr 2 is a protein containing 369 amino acids. It possesses four putative N-glycosylation sites and an intracellularly located target sequence for protein kinase A (PKA). The receptor is able to modulate several intracellular second-messenger systems. Inhibition of adenylate cyclase, activation of tyrosine phosphatase and phospholipase C, and intracellular Ca^{2+} mobilization have been described (Tomura et al. 1994).

sstr 5 contains 363 amino acids. The protein contains three putative N-glycosylation sites, three consensus sequences for PKA phosphorylation, and three target sequences for protein kinase C.

Pharmacologically, sstr 5 differs from the other sstrs in term of its higher affinity for somatostatin-28 (Patel and Srikant 1995). The receptor is coupled to adenylate cyclase and phospholipase C. Interestingly, no modification of phosphotyrosine phosphatase was found (Reardon et al. 1997). Somatostatin-28, but not somatostatin-14 or cortistatin, can induce ligand-dependent receptor internalization. In this context it is important to mention that most studies were performed in heterologous systems, while no information is available about the effects of the human somatostatin receptors on human cells.

Somatostatin Receptor Expression in Endocrine Gastroenteropancreatic Tumors

Somatostatin analogues are widely used for the treatment of endocrine gastroenteropancreatic (GEP) tumors. Early studies showed the presence of binding sites for somatostatin in these tissues (Reubi et al. 1987). Therefore, after cloning of the respective somatostatin receptor cDNAs it was of great interest to see which sstrs are expressed in these tissues. These studies were done using specific assays, including RT-PCR and in situ hybridization. The tumor types most often studied include gastrinomas, insulinomas, tumors responsible for the carcinoid syndrome, and functionally inactive tumors (Reubi et al. 1994; Vikic-Topic et al. 1995; Jonas et al. 1995; Kubota et al. 1995; John et al. 1996; Schaer et al. 1997, Jais et al. 1997; Wulbrand et al. 1998). sstr 1 is frequently found in gastrinomas and insulinomas, while its expression is reduced in carcinoid tumors and functionally inactive tumors. Receptor subtype 2 is present in almost all gastrinomas and insulinomas and in most carcinoid tumors and functionally inactive neoplasms. sstr 3 and 4 are rarely expressed in all four tumor types. sstr 5 is frequently present in gastrinomas and insulinomas, and less in carcinoid tumors and in functionally inactive neoplasms. It is important to mention that only two studies investigated all five somatostatin receptor subtypes in larger numbers of these tumors. In our study the expression frequency was statistically different for sstr 1 and 2 (Wulbrand et al. 1998). All data are carefully summarized in our paper. Thus, the reduced expression of sstr 5 in functionally inactive tumors could be of importance for the derailed growth regulation.

One of the most striking results was the extremely low expression of sstr 3 in these tumors. Is this an advantage for the tumor? The biological significance has not yet been elucidated. Interestingly, sstr 3 was shown to induce apoptosis via dephosphorylation-dependent conformation changes in p53 as well as via induction of Bax (Sharma et al. 1996).

Most gastrinomas, insulinomas, and carcinoid tumors expressed the IGF-1, the TGF-β1, and the TGF-β2 receptor. EGF receptor mRNAs were found in all gastrinomas and in only one insulinoma and carcinoid tumor each (Wulbrand et al. 1998). We did not detect any correlation between somatostatin receptor subtype expression and tumor localization or the presence/absence of metastases at the time of operation.

Treatment of Endocrine GEP Tumors with Somatostatin Analogues

Therapeutic strategies of endocrine GEP tumors follow two aims. First, hormone secretion must be reduced in order to control the clinical syndrome of hormone excess. Second, the tumor growth must be controlled.

Effects of Somatostatin Analogues on Hormone Secretion

Somatostatin analogues are very effective in controlling hormone secretion from endocrine GEP tumors. VIP release from VIPomas is normalized or significantly improved in 75% of patients. Both the reduced hormone release and a reduced intestinal fluid secretion reverse excessive diarrhea as the main symptom in patients with Verner-Morrison syndrome (Scarpignato 1995), and 90% of patients suffering from necrolytic migrating erythema due to a malignant glucagonoma and from flush, diarrhea, and bronchoconstriction as consequences of a carcinoid syndrome respond to octreotide therapy (Frankton and Bloom 1996; Ruszniewski et al. 1996). Interestingly, hormone secretion was normalized/reduced in only 40% of patients with carcinoid syndrome. In 1995, Harris and Redfern reviewed the available literature concerning the action of octreotide in patients with carcinoid syndromes. Data from 62 reports were summarized. All studies showed that octreotide is beneficial for these patients. Daily dosages of 0.15–0.2 mg/day reduced diarrhea and flushing in about 40% of patients. A maximal response was observed at daily dosages between 0.4 and 1 mg/day. Higher concentrations failed to improve the results. Comparable to our own data is the finding that 5-HIAA excretion is reduced to a lesser extent than the symptoms. The response to octreotide in insulinoma was variable. The peptide was able to reduce plasma insulin levels in 50% of patients with insulinoma (Boden 1989).

In contrast, gastric acid hypersecretion, ulcers, and diarrhea in patients with gastrinoma can be perfectly controlled by proton pump inhibitors, and there is no indication in such cases for somatostatin analogues (Arnold and Frank 1996).

Effects of Somatostatin Analogues on Tumor Growth

The second aim in treating endocrine GEP tumors is the control of tumor growth. Chemotherapy is not the first choice, since published data show unpredictable response rates, toxic side effects, and the lack of reliable parameters that could help to identify patients who might respond to the therapy. The respective protocols have recently been reviewed (Arnold and Frank 1995, 1996). There is good evidence that octreotide is able to reduce tumor growth at least in a subgroup of patients with endocrine GEP tumors. In one study 21 patients with metastatic endocrine GEP tumors (including gastrinomas, carcinoid syndrome, and functionally inactive tumors) were treated with 200 µg octreotide three times daily (Arnold et al. 1993). Tumor growth was documented by ultrasonography and CT. Five patients were considered responders, seven questionable responders, and nine did not respond. The most favorable response was growth arrest. An escape was observed in all but one responder. All responders showed reduced hormone secretion. Some patients had suppressed hormone levels although the tumor growth remained unaltered.

A second study evaluated the effectiveness of octreotide (200 µg three times daily) in patients with metastatic neuroendocrine GEP tumors (Arnold et al. 1996). Tumor growth was studied prior to treatment in all patients. This is of special importance, since tumor growth varies from patient to patient, and even in the same patient progression is variable and unpredictable. In the group of 52 patients with tumor progression prior to octreotide therapy, 16 (30%) responded with stabilization of tumor growth lasting from 3 to 48 months. Thirteen patients had stable disease during the observation period; 50% remained stable during therapy. In both groups no tumor regression was observed. Saltz et al. (1993) reported 52% responders among 32 patients, with maintainable stabilization of tumor growth for at least 2 months. There was no correlation between patient characteristics and the response pattern. In addition, single case reports documented even a regression of neuroendocrine GEP tumors during octreotide therapy (Clements and Elias 1985; Boden et al. 1986; Shepherd and Senator 1986; Wiedenmann et al. 1988). In conclusion, these data document antiproliferative effects of octreotide at least in subgroups of patients with neuroendocrine tumors. Clinical and biochemical characteristics of these subgroups are still unidentified.

Future Directions

Cloning of the five somatostatin receptors allows a better understanding of the physiology and pathophysiology of these proteins. It is now possible to study the regulation of expression, the intracellular trafficking, and the regulation of receptor proteins present in the cell membrane. Subtype-selective analogues can now be developed. It should be possible to create drugs that recognize only one somatostatin receptor subtype. In the case of sstr 2, such analogues have been designed (Yang et al. 1998). It is reasonable to speculate that such drugs could represent new tools for the treatment of endocrine GEP tumors. From our perspective, the sstr 3 is an interesting protein. This receptor is absent in these tumors. Of course, this could represent a biological advantage of the tumor, since sstr 3 can induce intracellular signals leading to apoptosis. It is not known whether the gene is mutated. On the other hand, its expression could be actively suppressed or defectively inactivated. In any case, it would be of special interest to determine whether this receptor is able to induce apoptosis in these tumors, as has been described in vitro. In this case, a re-expression of sstr 3 could be very helpful. We expect that the results of basic research will help to develop new important therapeutic aspects for the treatment of patients with neuroendocrine GEP tumors.

References

Arnold R, Frank M (1995) Systemic chemotherapy for endocrine tumors of the pancreas: recent advances. In: Mignon M, Jensen RT (eds) Endocrine tumors of the pancreas. Karger, Basel, pp 431–438

Arnold R, Frank M (1996) Gastrointestinal endocrine tumors: medical management. Baillieres Clin Gastroenterol 10:737–759

Arnold R, Neuhaus C, Benning R, Schwerk WB, Trautmann ME, Joseph K, Bruns C (1993) Somatostatin analog sandostatin and inhibition of tumor growth in patients with metastatic endocrine gastroenteropancreatic tumors. World J Surg 17:511–519

Arnold R, Trautmann ME, Creutzfeldt W, Benning R, Benning M, Neuhaus C, Jürgensen R, Stein K, Schäfer H, Bruns C, Dennler HJ (1996) Somatostatin analogue octreotide and inhibition of tumour growth in metastatic endocrine gastroenteropancreatic tumours. Gut 38:430–438

Boden G (1989) Glucagonomas and insulinomas. Gastrenterol Clin North Am 18:831–847

Boden G, Ryan IG, Eisenschmidt BL, Shelmet JJ, Owen OE (1986) Treatment of inoperable glucagonoma with long-acting somatostatin analogue SMS 201-995. N Engl J Med 314:1686–1689

Brazeau P, Vale W, Burgus R, Ling N, Butcher M, Rivier J, Guilleman R (1973) Hypothalamic polypeptide that inhibits the secretion of immunoreactive pituitary growth hormone. Science 179:77–79

Clements D, Elias E (1985) Regression of metastatic VIPoma with somatostatin analogue SMS 201-995. Lancet 1:874–875

de Lecea L, Criado JR, Propero-Garcia O, Gautvik KM, Schweitzer P, Danielson PE, Dunlop CLM, Siggins GR, Nenrksen SJ, Sutcliffe JG (1996) A cortical neuropeptide with neuronal depressant and sleep-modulating properties. Nature 381:242–245

Fehmann HC, Arnold R (1996) Molekularbiologie, Pharmakologie uns Signaltransduktion der fünf klonierten humanen Somatostatin Rezeptoren. Z Gastroenterol 34:767–774

Frankton S, Bloom SR (1996) Glucagonomas. Baillieres Clin Gastroenterol 10:697–705

Fukusumi S, Kitada C, Takekawa S, Sakamoto M, Miyamoto M, Hinuma S, Kitano K, Fujino M (1997) Identification and characterization of a novel human cortistatin-like peptide. Biochem Biophys Res Commun 232:157–163

Harris AG, Redfern JS (1995) Octreotide treatment of carcinoid syndrome: analysis of published dose-titration data. Aliment Pharmacol Ther 9:387–394

Jais P, Terris B, Ruszniewski P, Le Romancer M, Reyl-Desmars F, Vissuzaine C, Cadiot G, Mignon M, Lewin MJM (1997) Somatostatin receptor subtype gene expression in human endocrine gastroentero-pancreatic tumours. Eur J Clin Invest 27:639–644

John M, Meyerhof W, Richter D (1996) Positive somatostatin receptor scintigraphy correlates with the presence of somatostatin receptor subtype 2. Gut 38:33–39

Jonas S, John M, Boese-Landgraf J (1995) Somatostatin receptor subtypes in neuroendocrine tumor cell lines and tumor tissues. Langenbecks Arch Chir 380:90–95

Kubota A, Yamada Y, Kagimoto S, Shimatsu A, Imamura M, Tsuda K, Imura H, Seine S, Seino Y (1995) Identification of somatostatin receptor subtypes and an implication for the efficacy of somatostatin analogue SMS 201-995 in treatment of human endocrine tumors. J Clin Invest 93:1321–1325

Lamberts SWJ, Lely AJ, Herder WW, Hofland L (1996) Octreotide. N Engl J Med 334:246–254

Montminy MR, Goodman RH, Horovitch SJ, Habener JF (1984) Primary structure of the gene encoding rat prosomatostatin. Proc Natl Acad Sci USA 81:3337–3340

Patel Y, Srikant CB (1995) Subtype selectivity of peptide analogs for all five cloned human somatostatin receptors (hSSTR1-5). Endocrinology 135:2814–2817

Reardon DB, Dent P, Wood SL, Kong T, Sturgill TW (1997) Activation in vitro of somatostatin receptor subtypes 2, 3 or 4 stimulates protein tyrosine phosphatase activity in membranes from transfected ras transformed NIH 3T3 cells: coexpression with catalytically inactive SHP-2 blocks responsiveness. Mol Endocrinol 11:1062–1069

Reubi JC, Häcki W, Lamberts SWJ (1987) Hormone-producing gastrointestinal tumors contain a high density of somatostatin receptors. J Clin Endocrinol Metab 65:1127–1134

Reubi JC, Schaer JC, Waser B, Mengod G (1994) Expression and localization of somatostatin receptor SSTR1, SSTR2 and SSTR3 mRNAs in primary human tumors using in situ hybridization. Cancer Res 54:3455–3459

Ruszniewski P, Ducreux M, Chayvialle JA (1996) Treatment of carcinoid syndrome with the long-acting somatostatin analogue lanreotide: a prospective study in 39 patients. Gut 39:279–283

Saltz L, Trochanowsky G, Buckley M, Heffernan B, Niedzwicki D, Tao Y, Kelsen D (1993) Octreotide as an anti-neoplastic agent in the treatment of functional and non-functional neuroendocrine tumours. Cancer 72:244–248

Scarpignato C (1995) Somatostatin analogues in the management of endocrine tumors of the pancreas. In: Mignon M, Jensen RT (eds) Endocrine tumors of the pancreas. Karger, Basel, pp 385–414

Schaer JC, Waser B, Mengod G, Reubi JC (1997) Somatostatin receptor subtypes sstl, sst2, sst3, sst4, sst5 expression in human pituitary, gastroenteropancreatic and mammary tumors: comparison of MRNA analysis with receptor autoradiography. Int J Cancer 70:530–537

Sharma K, Patel YC, Srikant CB (1996) Subtype-selective induction of wild-type p53 and apoptosis, but not cell cycle arrest, by human somatostatin receptor 3. Mol Endocrinol 10:1688–1696

Shepherd JJ, Senator GB (1986) Regression of liver metastases in patient with gastrin-secreting tumour treated with SMS 201-995. Lancet 2:574

Tomura H, Okajima F, Akbar M, Abdul-Majid M, Sho K, Kondo Y (1994) Transfected human somatostatin receptor type 2, SSTR2, not only inhibits adenylate cyclase but also stimulates phospholipase C and Ca^{2+} mobilization. Biochem Biophys Res Commun 200:986–992

Vikic-Topic S, Raisch KP, Kvols LK, Vuk-Pavlovic S (1995) Expression of somatostatin receptor subtypes in breast carcinoma, carcinoid tumors and renal cell carcinoma. J Clin Endocrinol Metab 80:2974–2979

Wiedenmann B, Räth U, Rädsch R, Becker F, Kommereil B (1988) Tumour regression of an ileal carcinoid under treatment with the somatostatin analogue SMS 201-995. Klin Wochenschr 66:75–77

Wulbrand U, Wied M, Zöfel P, Göke B, Arnold R, Fehmann HC (1998) Growth factor receptor expression in human gastroenteropancreatic neuroendocrine tumours. Eur J Clin Invest 28:1038–1049

Yang L, Berk SC, Rohrer SP, Mosley RT, Guo L et al (1998) Synthesis and biological activities of potent peptidomimetics selective for somatostatin receptor subtype 2. Proc Natl Acad Sci USA 95:10836

The Significance of Somatostatin Analogues in the Antiproliferative Treatment of Carcinomas

R. Kath and K. Höffken

Klinik und Poliklinik für Innere Medizin II (Onkologie, Hämatologie, Endokrinologie, Stoffwechselerkrankungen), Friedrich-Schiller-Universität Jena, 07740 Jena, Germany

Abstract

Somatostatin is a cyclic tetradecapeptide hormone. It was initially isolated from bovine hypothalami. Somatostatin inhibits endocrine and exocrine secretion, as well as tumor cell growth, by binding to specific cell-surface receptors. Its potent inhibitory activity is limited, however, by its rapid enzymatic degradation and the consequently short plasma half-life. Octreotide is a short somatostatin analogue with increased duration of action compared with somatostatin. Preclinical studies have focused on the anticancer effects of octreotide and the related somatostatin analogues. In vitro, at nanomolar concentrations, these analogues inhibit the growth of tumor cells that express high-affinity somatostatin receptors. Accordingly, such analogues potently inhibit the growth of somatostatin receptor-positive tumors in various rodent models. The range of cancers susceptible to octreotide and related somatostatin analogues includes mammary, pancreatic, gastric, colorectal, prostate, thyroid, and lung carcinomas. Moreover, an indirect antiproliferative effect of somatostatin analogues is achievable in somatostatin receptor-negative tumors whose growth is driven by factors (e.g., gastrin, insulin-like growth factor-1) that become downregulated by somatostatin. The clinical effect of somatostatin analogues in terms of tumor response in cancer patients is a subject of controversy, however. Most responses have been seen in patients with pancreatic cancers.

Introduction

Three particular cyclo-octapeptide analogues, namely octreotide (SMS 201-995, Sandostatin), somatuline (BIM 23014), and vapreotide (RC-160), have been synthesized and investigated in depth. Octreotide exhibits a markedly increased stability in the circulation (plasma half-life ~2 h). It has been approved for use in the treatment of several malignancies.

A number of different somatostatin receptor subtypes have been identified and appear to be linked to a variety of signal transduction pathways, including tyrosine phosphatase, and stimulation of this pathway in receptor subtypes SSTR1 and SSTR2 has been shown to inhibit cell proliferation in vitro. Furthermore, increased detection of the SSTR2 subtype in peritumoral veins surrounding human colon cancer specimens suggest this may be a specific tumor-host interaction.

Activity of Somatostatin Analogues in Various Cancer Models

The somatostatin analogues octreotide, BIM 23014, and RC-160 have been extensively tested in vitro with regard to their antiproliferative properties. Because octreotide, BIM 23014, and RC-160 are structurally related, both the range of their biological activities and their potency are comparable, if not identical, in a number of endocrine and oncological models. Either animal or human cancer cell lines were used in proliferation assays. The extent of cell growth inhibition was determined by measuring parameters such as cell count, cell protein, or thymidine incorporation after exposure of the test cell lines to nanomolar concentrations of the analogues. A number of cell lines inhibited by somatostatin analogues were also shown to be somatostatin receptor positive. Thus, the antiproliferative action of the somatostatin analogues is obviously mediated by high-affinity somatostatin receptors on these tumor cells.

The growth of somatostatin receptor-negative cells lines, such as the human mammary cancer cell line MDA-MB-231, failed to be inhibited by even high concentrations ($1 \, \mu M$) of octreotide. Contradictory results were obtained with the pancreatic cancer cell line MIA PaCa-2 in vitro. For example, Gillespie et al. (1992) detected neither somatostatin receptors nor an effect of RC-160 on the growth of MIA Pa-Ca-2 cells. By contrast, Radulovic et al. (1993) found the same cell line both to be growth inhibited by RC-160 and to express binding sites for radiolabeled RC-160.

It has been shown that the combination of octreotide with other hormonal treatment (Weckbecker et al. 1994) in breast cancer cell lines and with cytokines (di Paolo et al. 1995) or 5-fluorouracil (Romani and Morris 1995) in colon cancer cell lines has synergistic effects.

In Vivo Activity of Somatostatin Analogues

The somatostatin analogues octreotide, BIM 23014, and RC-160 have been studied in various rodent cancer models, with special emphasis on human tumor xenotransplants in nude mice. The effect of these analogues was determined by recording the change in tumor volume during and after treatment. Only a few studies have addressed the inhibitory effect of somatostatin analogues on carcinogenesis or metastatic spread. The therapy with somatostatin analogues was often started when tumors were rather small. The somatostatin analogues were administered either by daily or twice-daily bolus injections or by continuous infusion using osmotic minipumps. The doses reported to be effective in the various models varied significantly, but there was a general tendency to use high-dose regimens such as 10 µg/kg/h (infusion) or 2.5 mg/kg (bolus injection).

Frequently, the outcome of somatostatin treatment has been related to the somatostatin receptor status of the tumors being treated. In contrast to the situation in vitro, where only somatostatin receptor-positive tumor cells are sensitive to somatostatin analogues, tumors without specific high-affinity somatostatin receptors can respond in vivo to treatment with somatostatin analogues. The initiation of cancer therapy with somatostatin analogues seems to be optimal when tumors express high levels of somatostatin receptors. However, tumors change their properties during progression. For example, prostate and breast cancers express receptors for androgens and estrogens, respectively, at an early stage, but they frequently become hormone insensitive in an advanced stage of the disease. Similarly, somatostatin receptors seem to be markers of a less malignant, more differentiated stage of a tumor.

The presence of specific receptors for somatostatin on a human breast cell line (MCF-7) was first reported by Setyono Han et al. (1987). Contradictory correlations between somatostatin receptor and sex-steroid receptors have been described. Reubi and Torhorst (1989) found a positive correlation between somatostatin receptors and steroid receptors in 36 tumors, but no correlation with these parameters was found by Prevost et al. (1992).

The presence of immunoreactive somatostatin was investigated by immunohistochemistry in 40 biopsies from breast cancer patients (Ciocca et al. 1990). Immunoreactivity was absent in normal mammary tissue and present in about 30% of the tumor samples. This presence was also detected in cultured cell lines. Human breast cancer cell lines (ZR-75, MDAMB-436, and MCF-7) were found to synthesize somatostatin detected by immunoreactivity assay in the culture media (Nelson et al. 1989).

Mammary Cancer

Studies In Vivo

The interest in studying the effects of somatostatin analogues in breast cancer models in vivo is due (a) to the detection of a high incidence of somatostatin receptor-positive mammary tumors (Reubi et al. 1990) and (b) early studies showing that the growth of human breast cancer cells in vitro is inhibited by the somatostatin analogues.

The growth of the human estrogen-dependent breast cancer cell line MCF-7 in nude mice was significantly retarded by twice-daily injections of octreotide (0.2 mg/kg), with tumor doubling time being increased from 13.2 days (control) to 19 days (octreotide). Similarly, BIM-23014 reduced the growth of MCF-7 tumors in a nude mouse subrenal capsule assay (Prevost et al. 1992). In the latter study a ligand cross-linking procedure was used to show that the tumors expressed binding sites for somatostatin-14 and BIM 23014.

Indirect effects may also play an important role in the treatment of mammary cancer with somatostatin analogues. Dimethylbenzanthracene (DMBA)-induced rat tumors are heterogeneous in somatostatin receptor expression, but they responded to continuous treatment with octreotide (0.01 mg/kg/h), in that the tumor multiplicity (number of tumors per animal) was reduced. This indicates that octreotide may be more active in the initial phase of tumorigenesis. Liebow et al.(1993) showed that RC-160 apparently reverses the development of malignancies initiated by local administration of DMBA. Conflicting results (inhibition and lack of inhibition) were obtained in the DMBA model with bolus injection of octreotide (Setyono Han et al. 1987; Bakker et al. 1990). MDA-MB-468 human breast tumors growing in nude mice provide another example of the indirect effects of octreotide. Mammary cancer frequently progresses from an estrogen-dependent, more benign form to an estrogen-independent, aggressive form. From the limited data obtained in models of estrogen-dependent mammary cancer (ZR-75–1, MCF-7, DMBA) and estrogen-independent cancer (MDA-MB-468), it appears that somatostatin analogues such as octreotide could be active for therapy of both types of breast cancer.

Clinical Studies

Twenty-four stage-IV breast cancer patients were enrolled in a phase-I safety/tolerability study of high-dose octreotide. Patients were enrolled in cohorts of four to six patients each and were treated with doses of 0.5–2.0 mg s.c. for 8 weeks. Patients having stable disease or a response to therapy were allowed to continue at either enrollment dose until disease progression occurred. Two patients had stable disease lasting 24 and 34 weeks; the latter patient had a 47% decrease in the volume of liver metastases, but did not have a response in bony lesions as assessed by bone scan (Novartis data on file).

One phase-II open-labeled trial enrolled patients with advanced estrogen receptor-negative breast cancer, and another trial enrolled patients with estrogen receptor-positive breast cancer. These patients received 2 mg octreotide three times a day (t.i.d.). Fifteen patients were entered with estrogen-negative disease; no responses occurred, but one patient had stable disease for >10 months. Seventeen patients with estrogen-positive disease entered; one partial response was observed (Novartis data on file).

Ingle et al. (1996) reported on patients with metastatic breast cancer and no prior systemic treatment who received 0.15 mg octreotide t.i.d. subcutaneously. They observed no objective responses. The median time to treatment failure was short at 57 days.

In 33 postmenopausal, previously untreated breast cancer patients Canobbio et al. (1995) found a significant synergistic reduction of plasma IGF-I concentrations following BIM 23014 and tamoxifen treatment; 12.5% of the patients exhibited a complete, 37.5% a partial remission. This effect of somatostatin analogues in combination with hormonal treatment might also be used for the adjuvant treatment of breast cancer (Pollak and Hankinson 1998).

Shiba et al. (1996) described successful treatment with octreotide (0.1 mg/day s.c.) in a patient with malignant hypercalcemia associated with advanced breast cancer who no longer responded to pamidronate.

Vennin et al. (1989) evaluated the effect of a long-acting somatostatin analogue (SMS 201-995) in 16 patients with advanced breast cancer. They administered 0.1 mg SMS 201-995 s.c. b.i.d. and found no objective response. Stolfi et al. (1990) treated ten patients with advanced breast cancer with 0.75 mg SMS i.m. b.i.d. for 10 days, followed by 0.5 mg i.m. b.i.d. for 5 days; three of the patients achieved a partial response.

Colorectal Cancer

Studies In Vivo

Smith and Solomon (1988) showed that twice-daily injections of 0.1 and 0.3 mg/kg somatostatin-14, dissolved in hydrolyzed gelatin to prolong absorption, induced significant inhibition of the growth of human colon adenocarcinomas in nude mice. Dy et al. (1992) found that continuous administration of octreotide at daily doses of 5–50 µg/kg caused a significant dose-related inhibition of the growth of human colorectal tumor xenotransplants. Long-term treatment with 50 µg/kg RC-160 twice a day inhibited the growth of liver metastases induced by intrasplenic injection of DHD/K12 colon adenocarcinoma cells into syngeneic BDIX rats. Since the growth of DHD/K12 cells was also inhibited in vitro, a direct somatostatin receptor-mediated effect can be assumed.

An indirect inhibitory effect of octreotide on tumor growth was apparently obtained with murine colonic adenocarcinoma cells CT-26. Cell proliferation in vitro was not inhibited by octreotide, but the growth of CT-26 tumors in mice was greatly suppressed, indicating an inhibitory effect of octreotide on growth factors and hormones stimulating CT-26 tumor growth in vivo.

There are several pieces of evidence from animal models which support the role of octreotide in the treatment and/or prevention of hepatic metastases from colorectal adenocarcinoma. Nott et al. (1989) demonstrated that subcutaneous administration of octreotide significantly inhibited the growth and development of liver metastases following intraportal injection of colon carcinoma Walker cells.

A study by Stewart et al. (1994) used a hepatic metastases model in athymic nude mice following intrasplenic injection of the colonic carcinoma cell line C170. Treatment with high-dose octreotide for 28 days significantly reduced the number and weight of hepatic metastases (Fig. 1).

Another study (van Eijck et al. 1994) was designed to test the hypothesis that response to octreotide was correlated to the presence of somatostatin receptors in tumors, which appears to be the case with endocrine tumors. Two models of hepatic metastases were established by intraportal injection of somatostatin receptor-positive pancreatic tumor cells or somatostatin receptor-negative colonic tumor cells. In this model, octreotide significantly inhibited the growth and development of somatostatin receptor-positive tumor cells in the liver but had no effect on receptor-negative cells. This finding occurred in the absence of any de-

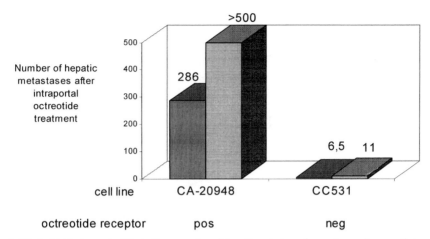

Fig. 1. Effect of high-dose octreotide in the prevention of hepatic metastases from colon carcinoma cells in nude mice. (From Stewart et al. 1994)

tectable difference in serum levels of growth hormone, prolactin, and IGF between control and octreotide-treated rats, consistent with a re-ceptor-dependent effect. This suggests that octreotide may be effective in the treatment of somatostatin receptor-positive hepatic metastases following their detection by somatostatin receptor scintigraphy. Both of these studies show that octreotide is an effective treatment of hepa-tic metastases in experimental models and suggest that the effect is mediated through specific somatostatin receptors.

Clinical Studies

Goldberg et al. (1995) performed a phase-III evaluation of octreotide in the treatment of patients with asymptomatic advanced colon carci-noma in which 260 patients without symptoms related to colon can-cer were randomized to receive 0.150 mg t.i.d. of octreotide or place-bo s.c. They found no clinical benefit (time to progression, survival) for octreotide (Fig. 2).

Cascinu et al. (1997) recently reported on the inhibition of cell ki-netics and serum insulin growth factor I levels by octreotide in colorec-tal cancer patients. Seventy-five patients were randomized to be treated either with octreotide (0.2 mg) for 2 weeks prior to surgery or with the usual medication. Samples of tumor tissue were taken at endoscopy and at surgery; thus, growth factors and cell kinetics could be assessed prior to and after treatment (Table 1). Similar results on kinetic modifications

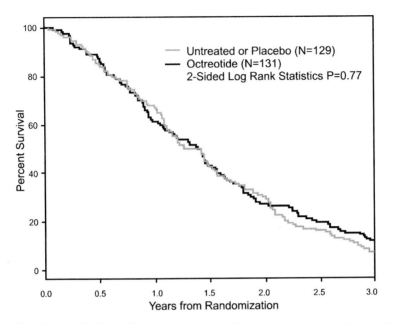

Fig. 2. Survival of patients with asymptomatic advanced colon carcinoma treated with octreotide or placebo. (From Goldberg et al. 1995)

Table 1. Effect of preoperative octreotide treatment on tumor cell kinetics in colorectal cancer patients[a]

		Percentage of S-phase fraction		
		A+ Endoscopy	A+ Operation	p value
Thymidine-labeling index	Control group (n=31)	19.65±3.61	17.55±2.15	NS
	Octreotide-treated patients (n=32)	17.85±5.65	3.4±1.16	0.0001
Flow cytometry	Control group (n=38)	20.97±10.21	21.93±7.92	NS
	Octreotide-treated patients (n=37)	26.98±14.17	21.53±8.08	0.013

[a] Values are expressed as means ±SEM, and n=number of evaluable patients.

were reported by Stewart et al. (1995). Cascinu et al. (1995) also reported on a significant survival benefit in advanced colorectal carcinoma treated with low-dose octreotide (Fig. 3).

The therapeutic potential of octreotide in the treatment of liver metastasis was analyzed by Davies et al. (1996). Investigating several studies, they found poor tumor responses in advanced gastrointestinal cancer.

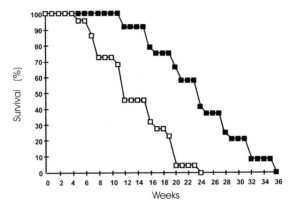

Fig. 3. Survival curves comparing patients with colorectal cancer treated with octreotide (■, $n=24$) or best supportive care (□, $n=22$). There is a statistically significant difference between the two arms. Mantel-Cox (log-rank), $p=0.001$. (Modified from Cascinu et al. 1995)

Pancreatic Cancer

Studies In Vivo

Hajri et al. (1991) showed that octreotide significantly retarded the growth of rat pancreatic acinar tumors over a 15-day treatment period. Using receptor autoradiography, somatostatin receptors were detected on this tumor. Octreotide treatment did not down-regulate the somatostatin receptors of the tumors.

The growth of MIA PaCA-2 tumors (derived from a human pancreatic cancer cell line) was dose-dependently inhibited in nude mice by twice-daily injections of octreotide (250 and 2500 µg/kg). Correspondingly, microcapsules of RC-160 releasing 25 µg/day significantly inhibited tumor growth in nude mice bearing MIA PaCa-2 tumors (Radulovic et al. 1993).

Estrogen and androgen receptors have been demonstrated in some pancreatic cancers, and antiestrogen and LHRH-agonist treatment have been reported to be beneficial in a few patients. Since somatostatin has a major effect on the hormone secretion of the pancreas, and in view of the poor prognosis and the lack of effective alternative treatments, somatostatin analogues have been proposed as a therapeutic option for pancreatic cancer. Production and expression of transforming growth factor (TGF) have been demonstrated by human pancreatic cancer cells. TGF is 10–100 times more potent than epidermal growth factor (EGF) in its effect on cellular proliferation and acts through the EGF receptor. Overexpression of the EGF receptor has also been clearly demonstrated in human pancreatic cancer cell lines. Here, TGF binds to the EGF receptor and acts as a superagonist autocrine growth regulator.

The action of TGF has therefore been strongly implicated in the growth of pancreatic cancer cells, and somatostatin has been shown to interfere with the activity of EGF and EGF receptors. In other studies, somatostatin has been shown to stimulate dephosphorylation of membrane receptors, which have an antiproliferative effect in MIA PaCa-2-cell lines. Further, pancreatic cancer tumor models have been reported to respond to somatostatin analogues. Tumor shrinkage and reduction in growth rates have been demonstrated.

Clinical studies

Büchler et al. (1994) reported the results of a phase-II trial of octreotide (2 mg t.i.d. s.c.) in the treatment of advanced pancreatic adenocarcinoma in 49 patients. All patients had previously undergone surgery or radiation therapy. A total of 45 patients were evaluable, and the median time to disease progression in this group was 4.9 months. The median survival was 5.9 months. Thirteen patients had stable progression at a median of 12 weeks, and one patient even experienced no further disease progression over a period of 24 weeks. Patients tolerated the high doses of octreotide well, and no major adverse events or study drop-out occurred.

Ebert et al. (1994) reported on the use of both high- and low-dose octreotide in the treatment of pancreatic cancer stage-III ($n = 13$) and stage-IV ($n = 9$) patients. Low-dose octreotide (0.1 mg t.i.d. s.c.) was doubled in cases where a 25% increase in tumor size was noted on CT scans over an 8-week period.

A further 12 patients with advanced pancreatic carcinoma, stage III ($n = 3$) and stage IV ($n = 9$), were treated with a high-dose octreotide regimen. This consisted of 0.1 mg s.c. t.i.d. for the first week, 0.5 mg for the second week, 1 mg for the third week, and finally 2 mg from the fourth week on. Tumor response was assessed by CT scan, ultrasonography, and measurement of tumor markers at 3 weeks, and then monthly after 2 months. Median survival for the low-dose group was 3 months. No decrease in pain was noted. Median survival for the high-dose group was 6 months. The increased survival in the high-dose group and the beneficial effects on quality of life and disease progression led the authors to conclude that high-dose octreotide represents a promising and well-tolerated therapy for advanced pancreatic cancer.

Rosenberg et al. (1995) reported on low-dose octreotide (0.1 mg) and tamoxifen (10 mg b.i.d.) in the treatment of adenocarcinoma of the pancreas. In their study, patients with unresectable or resected but metastasized carcinomas had an apparently increased survival of 12 months (Fig. 4).

Cascinu et al. (1995) reported on a randomized trial of octreotide versus best supportive care in 107 patients with various advanced gastrointestinal cancers; 32 patients (16 controls) had pancreatic cancer. Patients received either 0.2 mg octreotide t.i.d., 5 days a week, or best supportive care only. There was a significant survival benefit for the entire group of octreotide-treated patients. For the subgroup of pancreatic cancer patients as well, there was a statistically ($p=0.001$) relevant survival benefit (seven versus two patients had stable disease) (Fig. 5). A summary of the clinical studies on the use of octreotide in pancreatic cancer is presented in Table 2.

Recently, a case report appeared (Sulkowski et al. 1997) of a distal bile duct carcinoma treated with octreotide for 6 months. The patient showed complete tumor regression following treatment with 6 mg daily. Two years after the first diagnosis the patient is doing well and has no signs of recurrence.

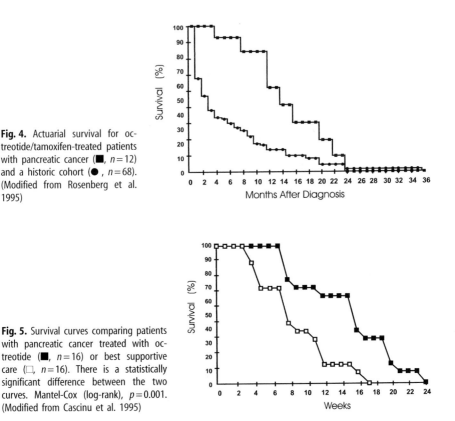

Fig. 4. Actuarial survival for octreotide/tamoxifen-treated patients with pancreatic cancer (■, $n=12$) and a historic cohort (●, $n=68$). (Modified from Rosenberg et al. 1995)

Fig. 5. Survival curves comparing patients with pancreatic cancer treated with octreotide (■, $n=16$) or best supportive care (□, $n=16$). There is a statistically significant difference between the two curves. Mantel-Cox (log-rank), $p=0.001$. (Modified from Cascinu et al. 1995)

Table 2. Summary of clinical studies on the use of octreotide in treating pancreatic cancer (*b.i.d.* twice daily, *t.i.d.* three times daily, *s.c.* subcutaneously)

Study population	Octreotide dose	Duration of treatment	Results	Reference
49 patients with advanced pancreatic adenocarcinoma	2 mg t.i.d. s.c.	Until disease progression/death	Median survival time was 5.9 months (3 months normally). Thirteen patients had stable disease at 12 weeks, one patient had stable disease at 24 weeks. No patient dropped out due to adverse events	Büchler et al. (1994)
Study I: 22 patients with advanced pancreatic cancer	0.1 mg t.i.d. s.c.	Until disease progression/death	Median survival was 3 months (no different from normal) and three patients had stable disease at 2 months. Mean survival was 6 months.	Ebert et al. (1994)
Study II: 12 patients with advanced pancreatic cancer	0.1–2 mg t.i.d. s.c.	Until disease progression/death	Median survival was 3 months (no different from normal) and three patients had stable disease at 2 months. Mean survival was 6 months.	Ebert et al. (1994)
12 patients with ductal pancreatic cancer; 68 untreated patients were controls	0.1 mg t.i.d. s.c. plus 10 mg b.i.d. orally	Until disease progression	One-year survival 59% as compared with 16% in the control group	Rosenberg et al. (1995)
32 patients with pancreatic cancer, 16 treated with octreotide and 16 with best supportive care only	0.2 mg t.i.d. 5 days a week or best supportive care only	Until disease progression	Significant response difference in favor of octreotide, seven vs two patients with stable disease	Cascinu et al. (1995)

Table 3. Synopsis of clinical trials including patients with advanced pancreatic cancer testing octreotide and LHRH analogues (*CR* complete remission, *PR* partial remission, *NC* no change in disease, *LHRH* luteinizing hormone-releasing hormone, *GNRH* gonadotropin-releasing hormone, *n.e.* not evaluable)

Agent	Treatment design	No. of patients evaluable for response	No. of responses			Median survival (months)	Reference
			CR	PR	NC		
Somatostatin analogues	3×200 µg/day octreotide	16			3	2	Klijn et al. (1990)
	3×100 µg/day octreotide	22			3	4	Friess et al. (1993)
	3×2000 g/day octreotide	10			4	6	Frieß et al. (1993)
	250–1000 µg/day BIM 23014	18		1	6	3	Canobbio et al. (1992)
	3×200 µg/day octreotide, 5 days/week	16			7	5	Cascinu et al. (1995)
	Control group: best supportive care	16			2	2.7	Cascinu et al. (1995)
LHRH analogues	3.6 mg goserelin q 4 weeks	10			8	7.5	Andrén-Sandberg (1989)
	D-Trp-6-LHRH days 1–7: 1 mg day 8 until PD: 100 µg	17		1	12	7.2	Gonzalez Barcena et al. (1989)
	Group A: 3.6 mg goserelin q 4 weeks	15			3	7.4	Sperti et al. (1992)
	Group B: no therapy	18			3	4.4	Sperti et al. (1992)
	1.2 mg buserelin	36			10	5	Frieß et al. (1992)
	3.6 mg goserelin q 4 weeks	7			n.e.	n.e.	Allegretti et al. (1993)
LHRH (GNRH) analogues plus somatostatin analogues	100 µg octreotide t.i.d. plus 1 mg/day leuprolide s.c.	21			5	4	Suri et al. (1991)
	3×250 µg/day BIM 23014 plus 3.75 mg Decapeptyl R q 4 weeks	38			n.e.	6	Huguier et al. (1992)
	Control group	43			n.e.	4.3	Huguier et al. (1992)

In a bicentric phase-II study, we treated 20 patients with locally advanced or metastatic pancreatic cancer with a combination of high-dose continuous-infusion octreotide (6 mg/day) and gemcitabine (days 1, 8, 15: 1 g/m^2, repeat day 28). The treatment was generally well tolerated. Response consisted of one PR, ten NC, and five PD among 16 evaluable patients (Kath et al. 1998). Several studies have been performed with a combination of LHRH analogues and somatostatin analogues in patients with pancreatic cancer. A synopsis of these is given in Table 3.

Recently, the results of a study of the long-acting octreotide SMS pa LAR in pancreatic cancer were presented at the 34th Annual Meeting of the Society for Clinical Oncology (Roy et al. 1998; ASCO 1998). In this randomized, double-blind, placebo-controlled phase-III trial, continuous-infusion 5-FU (225, mg/m^2 per day for 8 weeks) was given in both treatment arms, followed by a 1-week rest. Patients were cycled on a 9-week schedule unless significant toxicity occurred. Patients were randomized to receive either SMS pa LAR or placebo. At the interim analysis, 284 were enrolled and 281 had received at least one dose of study medication. One complete (SMS arm) and two partial remissions (one SMS, one placebo) were observed. The median survival of SMS-treated patients was 22.6 weeks (95% confidence interval 18.1–27.7) versus 21.6 weeks in the placebo arm (95% confidence interval 17.9–28.3) $p = 0.649$. There were no toxic deaths attributed to 5-FU or to SMS pa LAR. Although SMS pa LAR was safe and well tolerated, it had no activity in adenocarcinoma of the pancreas. A sister trial of SMS pa LAR vs placebo, in which no chemotherapy was used, revealed a median survival of 16.4 weeks (95% confidence interval 13.9–19.6) in a similar patient population. 5-FU remains one of the most active and well-tolerated agents in the treatment of pancreatic cancer (Pederzoli et al. 1998).

Gastric Cancer

The proliferation of normal gastric epithelial mucosa is controlled by a number of hormones and growth factors. The first indication that gastrin, a polypeptide hormone which is trophic for normal gastrointestinal epithelial cells, was implicated in the control of gastric mucosal growth was the observation that removal of the source of gastrin by antrectomy led to gastric mucosal atrophy, which was reversible by pentagastrin administration. Conversely, the hypergastrinemia associated with Zollinger-Ellison syndrome leads to gastric mucosal hyperplasia.

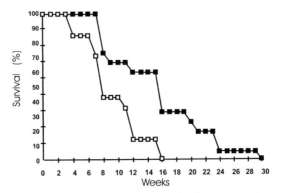

Fig. 6. Survival curves comparing patients with stomach cancer treated with octreotide (■, $n = 15$) or best supportive care (□, $n = 14$). There is a statistically significant difference between the two curves. Mantel-Cox (log-rank), $p = 0.003$. (Modified from Cascinu et al. 1995)

Gastrin is also known to promote the growth of gastric cancer cells in vitro (Watson et al. 1988) and to stimulate the growth of 50% of gastric carcinoma xenografts in vivo (Baldwin and Whitehead 1994). Despite this wealth of experimental evidence supporting mitogenic stimulation of gastric tumors in vitro and in vivo, there appears to be no evidence that it plays a role in the development of gastric adenocarcinoma. The finding that serum gastrin levels may be elevated in other types of cancer, e.g., colon cancer, is consistent with the hypothesis that gastrin and other gut hormones may act as autocrine growth factors in gastrointestinal cancer. Both transforming growth factor a (TGF-a) and insulin-like growth factor-I (IGF-I) can promote gastric cancer cell line growth in vitro with an additive mitogenic response, suggesting an independent effect at different receptors.

So far, only a few clinical data have been accumulated to support the preclinical observations. The above-mentioned study by Cascinu et al. (1995) also included gastric cancer patients. Patients treated with octreotide had a statistically significant survival benefit (Fig. 6).

Small Cell Lung Carcinoma

Despite the clinical relevance of small cell lung carcinomas (SCLC) and the unambiguous demonstration of somatostatin receptor expression by SCLC, effects of somatostatin analogues on lung cancer have not received much attention at the preclinical level. Bogden et al. (1990) treated four human SCLCs growing in athymic nude mice with BIM 23014. This somatostatin analogue was administered b.i.d. at an ultra high dose (25 mg/kg), either on the side opposite the tumor or as an infusion around the tumor. All tumors responded. In particular, the perilesional administration of BIM 23014 led to a potent inhibition of tumor growth. Tumors such as NCI-H345 SCLC responded exclusively to the perilesional regimen, which might indicate that only high concentrations of the analogue at the tumor site can exert significant tumor growth-inhibitory effects. This cell line was somatostatin receptor positive, suggesting direct effects of BIM 23014 on tumor growth. However, other SCLC cell lines (LX-1 and NCI-N417) which responded in vivo expressed only low levels of somatostatin receptors. Accordingly, indirect effects may play an important role in the antitumor action of somatostatin analogues. Human small-cell lung cancer exhibits various neuroendocrine features and may have the same embryological origins as APUD cells.

Rieu et al. (1993) reported a paradoxical effect of octreotide on the ectopic secretion of corticotropin in two cases of SCLC, leading to an increase in ACTH and cortisol plasma levels. The authors had no explanation for this effect. Results of studies demonstrating a potential clinical benefit of somatostatin analogues are not available.

Prostate Cancer

It has been suggested that somatostatin analogues may be useful for the therapy of prostate cancer. However, only a small number of studies support this concept. The somatostatin octapeptide analogue DC-13-135, which was given at a daily dose of 100 µg/kg, reduced the weight of R-3327 rat prostate tumors by 41%. Using the same tumor model, Siegel et al. (1988) evaluated octreotide effects. Treatment was started when tumors were already rather large (700 mm^3), and tumor growth was followed by means of magnetic resonance imaging. After a 3-week treatment period with octreotide (100 µg/kg b.i.d.) tumor growth was inhibited by 42%. An interruption of treatment led to regrowth of the tumor.

Patients with prostate cancer usually respond to hormonal manipulation involving androgen deprivation using either medical or surgical castration. After a variable period of response, most patients with advanced metastatic prostate cancer develop progressive disease. Various prognostic factors have been implicated in determining the eventual outcome of the disease. High prolactin levels have been correlated with a poor prognosis, and raised GH levels have been linked to an increased metastatic potential of prostate cancer.

Recently, the role of somatostatin analogues in complete antiandrogen treatment in patients with prostate cancer has been investigated (Vainas et al. 1997). In an open, controlled study the efficacy of octreotide plus androgen blockade was compared with that of androgen blockade alone. Response rates and survival were similar in both groups, but disease-free survival was longer with combined treatment.

Thyroid Cancer

Ain and Taylor (1994) reported both proliferative and antiproliferative effects of octreotide on human thyroid carcinoma cell lines. They stated that this discordant action of octreotide may be explained by differential receptor binding.

The effect of octreotide on the growth and invasion of differentiated thyroid cancer cells was studied by Hoelting et al. (1996), who found that there was a growth inhibition in vitro but not in vivo. Invasion was less affected than growth, as shown by the MTT as a growth assay and the Matrigel as an invasion assay.

Patients with differentiated thyroid carcinoma may be treated with thyroxine in order to inhibit the release of TSH. Maini et al. (1994) demonstrated that octreotide used in combination with thyroxine potentiates the suppression of TSH levels following radioiodine scanning.

O'Byrne et al. (1996) analyzed four patients with medullary thyroid carcinoma treated with octreotide. In one patient, treatment resulted in a 30% drop in calcitonin levels within 90 min, which was maintained for 6 h, suggesting the presence of functional somatostatin receptors. Long-term treatment did not reduce serum calcitonin or CEA. In a second patient, calcitonin dropped by 24%. No change in calcitonin was seen in patients 3 and 4.

Lupoli et al. (1996) studied the efficacy and tolerability of octreotide and interferon in eight patients with medullary thyroid carcinoma. A maximum decrease in calcitonin levels was reached after 1 month in two patients and after 3 months in four patients. Calcitonin levels subsequently increased but did not reach pretherapy values. No significant change in the size of metastases was observed.

Mure et al. (1995) also found a lack of efficacy in patients with Cushing's syndrome and metastatic medullary thyroid carcinoma. They described two patients who received octreotide (0.3 mg/day) for 6 and 15 days, respectively. In both patients, Cushing's syndrome could be cured by only adrenalectomy.

Raue et al. (1995) reported on eight patients treated with octreotide (doses of 0.1–1 mg/day) who suffered from metastasized medullary carcinoma. Two of the eight patients had a remission with respect to the tumor markers calcitonin and CEA, lasting 10 and 12 months, respectively. One patient experienced remission of a lymph node metastasis.

Conclusion

Somatostatin analogues represent a promising approach not only to the treatment of neuroendocrine tumors but also in several cancers. The advantages include a wide range of inhibitory and antiproliferative actions. The efficacy of somatostatin analogues has been proven in a variety of preclinical studies. However, the tumor response in clinical cancer studies remains uncertain.

References

Ain KB, Taylor KD (1994) Somatostatin analogs affect proliferation of human thyroid carcinoma cell lines in vitro. J Clin Endocrinol Metab 78:1097–1102

Allegretti A, Lionetto R, Saccomanno S, Paganuzzi M, Onetto M, Martinoli C, Rollandi G, Marugo M, Fazzuoli L, Pugliese V (1993) LH-RH analogue treatment in adenocarcinoma of the pancreas: a phase II study. Gruppo Ligure per lo Studio del Pancreas. Oncology 50:77–80

Andrén-Sandberg Å (1989) Androgen influence on exocrine pancreatic cancer. Int J Pancreatol 4:363–369

ASCO (1998) Final Program Announcement. ASCO's Thirty-fourth Annual Meeting, Los Angeles Convention Center, Los Angeles, California. Proc ASCO 17

Bakker GH, Setyono Han B, Foekens JA, Portengen H, van Putten WL, de Jong FH, Lamberts SW, Reubi JC, Klijn JG (1990) The somatostatin analog Sandostatin (SMS201-995) in treatment of DMBA-induced rat mammary tumors. Breast Cancer Res Treat 17:23–32

Baldwin GS, Whitehead RH (1994) Gut hormones, growth and malignancy. Baillieres Clin Endocrinol Metab 1:8

Bogden AE, Taylor JE, Moreau JP, Coy DH, LePage DJ (1990) Response of human lung tumor xenografts to treatment with a somatostatin analogue (Somatuline). Cancer Res 14:50

Büchler M, Sulkowski U, Pederzoli P, Arnold R, Dinse P, Mietlowski W, Israeli R (1994) A phase II study of octreotide (SMS) in advanced pancreatic cancer. Proc Am Soc Clin Oncol 13:214 (abstr 642)

Canobbio L, Boccardo F, Cannata D, Gallotti P, Epis R (1992) Treatment of advanced pancreatic carcinoma with the somatostatin analogue BIM 23014. Preliminary results of a pilot study. Cancer 69:648–650

Canobbio L, Cannata D, Miglietta L, Boccardo F (1995) Somatuline (BIM 23014) and tamoxifen treatment of postmenopausal breast cancer patients: clinical activity and effect on insulin-like growth factor-I (IGF-I) levels. Anticancer Res 15:2687–2690

Cascinu S, Del FE, Catalano G (1995) A randomised trial of octreotide vs best supportive care only in advanced gastrointestinal cancer patients refractory to chemotherapy. Br J Cancer 71:97–101

Cascinu S, Del Ferro E, Grianti C, Ligi M, Ghiselli R, Foglietti G, Saba V, Lungarotti F, Catalano G (1997) Inhibition of tumor cell kinetics and serum insulin growth factor I levels by octreotide in colorectal cancer patients. Gastroenterology 3:113

Ciocca DR, Puy LA, Fasoli LC, Tello O, Aznar JC, Gago FE, Papa SI, Sonego R (1990) Corticotropin-releasing hormone, luteinizing hormone-releasing hormone, growth hormone-releasing hormone, and somatostatin-like immunoreactivities in biopsies from breast cancer patients. Breast Cancer Res Treat 15:3

Davies N, Cooke TG, Jenkins SA (1996) Therapeutic potential of octreotide in the treatment of liver metastases. Anticancer Drugs 7 [Suppl]:1

di Paolo A, Bocci G, Innocenti F, Agen C, Nardini D, Danesi R, del Tacca M (1995) Inhibitory effect of the somatostatin analogue SMS 201-995 and cytokines on the proliferation of human colon adenocarcinoma cell lines. Pharmacol Res 32:135–139

Dy DY, Whitehead RH, Morris DL (1992) SMS 201-995 inhibits in vitro and in vivo growth of human colon cancer. Cancer Res 52:917–923

Ebert M, Friess H, Berger HG, Büchler MW (1994) Role of octreotide in the treatment of pancreatic cancer. Digestion 55:48–51

Frank Raue K, Raue F, Ziegler R (1995) Therapy of metastatic medullary thyroid gland carcinoma with the somatostatin analog octreotide. Med Klin 90:63–66

Frieß H, Büchler M, Beglinger C, Weber A, Kunz J, Fritsch K, Dennler HJ, Berger HG (1993) Low-dose octreotide treatment is not effective in patients with advanced pancreatic cancer. Pancreas 8:540–545

Frieß H, Büchler M, Ebert M, Malfertheiner P, Dennler HJ, Berger HG (1993) Treatment of advanced pancreatic cancer with high-dose octretide. Int J Pancreatology 14:290–291

Frieß H, Büchler M, Kruger M, Berger HG (1992) Treatment of duct carcinoma of the pancreas with the LH-RH analogue buserelin. Pancreas 7:516–521

Gillespie J, Poston GJ, Schachter M, Guillou PJ (1992) Human pancreatic cancer cell lines do not express receptors for somatostatin. Br J Cancer 66:483–487

Goldberg RM, Moertel CG, Wieand HS, Krook JE, Schutt AJ, Veeder MH, Mailliard JA, Dalton RJ (1995) A phase III evaluation of a somatostatin analogue (octreotide) in the treatment of patients with asymptomatic advanced colon carcinoma. North Central Cancer Treatment Group and the Mayo Clinic. Cancer 76:961–966

Gonzalez Barcena D, Ibarra Olmos MA, Garcia Carrasco F, Gutierrez Samperio C, Comaru Schally AM, Schally AV (1989) Influence of D-Trp-6-LH-RH on the survival time in patients with advanced pancreatic cancer. Biomed Pharmacother 43:313–317

Hajri A, Bruns C, Marbach P, Aprahamian M, Longnecker DS, Damge C (1991) Inhibition of the growth of transplanted rat pancreatic acinar carcinoma with octreotide. Eur J Cancer 27:10

Hoelting T, Duh QY, Clark OH, Herfarth C (1996) Somatostatin analog octreotide inhibits the growth of differentiated thyroid cancer cells in vitro, but not in vivo. J Clin Endocrinol Metab 81:2638–2641

Huguier M, Samama G, Testart J, Mauban S, Fingerhut A, Nassar J, Houry S, Jaeck D, De Mestier P, Favre JP (1992) Treatment of adenocarcinoma of the pancreas with somatostatin and gonadoliberin (luteinizing hormone-releasing hormone). The French Associations for Surgical Research. Am J Surg 164:348–353

Kath R, Höffken K, Raida M, Haus U, Schneider O, Schmiegel W, Graeven U (1998) Phase II trial of high-dose continuous octreotide infusion and gemcitabine in advanced pancreatic cancer. Ann Hematol 77 [Suppl]:S48

Ingle JN, Kardinal CG, Suman VJ, Krook JE, Hatfield AK (1996) Octreotide as first-line treatment for women with metastatic breast cancer. Invest New Drugs 14:235–237

Klijn JG, Hoff AM, Planting AS, Verweij J, Kok T, Lamberts SW, Portengen H, Foekens JA (1990) Treatment of patients with metastatic pancreatic and gastrointestinal tumours with the somatostatin analogue Sandostatin: a phase II study including endocrine effects. Br J Cancer 62:627–630

Liebow C, Crean DH, Schally AV, Mang TS (1993) Peptide analogues alter the progression of premalignant lesions, as measured by Photofrin fluorescence. Proc Natl Acad Sci USA 1:5

Lupoli G, Cascone E, Arlotta F, Vitale G, Celentano L, Salvatore M, Lombardi G (1996) Treatment of advanced medullary thyroid carcinoma with a combination of recombinant interferon alpha-2b and octreotide. Cancer 1:5

Maini CL, Sciuto R, Tofani A (1994) TSH suppression by octreotide in differentiated thyroid carcinoma. Clin Endocrinol (Oxf) 40:335–339

Mure A, Gicquel C, Abdelmoumene N, Tenenbaum F, Francese C, Travagli JP, Gardet P, Schlumberger M (1995) Cushing's syndrome in medullary thyroid carcinoma. J Endocrinol Invest 18:180–185

Nelson J, Cremin M, Murphy RF (1989) Synthesis of somatostatin by breast cancer cells and their inhibition by exogenous somatostatin and Sandostatin. Br J Cancer 59:5

Nott DM, Baxter JY, Grime JS, Day DW, Cooke TG, Jenkins SA (1989) Effects of a somatostatin analogue (SMS 201-995) on the growth and development of hepatic tumour derived by intraportal injection of Walker cells in the rat. Br J Surg 76:11

O'Byrne KJ, O'Hare N, Sweeney E, Freyne PJ, Cullen MJ (1996) Somatostatin and somatostatin analogues in medullary thyroid carcinoma. Nucl Med Commun 17:810–816

Pederzoli P, Maurer U, Vollmer K, Büchler M, Kjaeve J, Van Cutsem E et al (1998) Phase 3 trial of SMS 201-995 pa LAR (SMS pa LAR) vs. placebo in unresectable stage II, III and IV pancreatic cancer. Proc. 34th Annual Meeting American Society of Clinical Oncology (ASCO), May 16–19, Los Angeles, Calif., 17:257a (Abstr)

Pollak M, Hankinson S (1998) Biology of breast cancer risk and prognosis. Adjuvant Ther Prim Breast Cancer 34 [Suppl 1]:10

Prevost G, Lanson M, Thomas F, Veber N, Gonzalez W, Beaupain R, Starzec A, Bogden A (1992) Molecular heterogeneity of somatostatin analogue BIM-23014C receptors in human breast carcinoma cells using the chemical cross-linking assay. Cancer Res 15:4

Radulovic S, Comaru Schally AM, Milovanovic S, Schally AV (1993) Somatostatin analogue RC-160 and LH-RH antagonist SB-75 inhibit growth of MIA PaCa-2 human pancreatic cancer xenografts in nude mice. Pancreas 8:1

Reubi JC, Krenning E, Lamberts SW, Kvols L (1990) Somatostatin receptors in malignant tissues. J Steroid Biochem Mol Biol 37:1073–1077

Reubi JC, Torhorst J (1989) The relationship between somatostatin, epidermal growth factor, and steroid hormone receptors in breast cancer. Cancer 15:6

Rieu M, Rosilio M, Richard A, Vannetzel JM, Kuhn JM (1993) Paradoxical effect of somatostatin analogues on the ectopic secretion of corticotropin in two cases of small cell lung carcinoma. Horm Res 39:207–212

Romani R, Morris DL (1995) SMS 201.995 (Sandostatin) enhances in-vitro effects of 5-fluorouracil in colorectal cancer. Eur J Surg Oncol 21:27–32

Rosenberg L, Barkun AN, Denis MH, Pollak M (1995) Low dose octreotide and tamoxifen in the treatment of adenocarcinoma of the pancreas. Cancer 75:23–28

Roy A, Jacobs A, Bukowsky R, Cunningham D, Hamm J, Schlag PM, Rosen P, Francois E, Finley G, Lipton A (1998) Phase III trial of SMS 201–995 pa LAR (SMS PA LAR) and continuous infusion (ci) 5-FU in unresectable stage II, III, and IV pancreatic cancer. Proc. 34th Annual Meeting, American Society of Clinical Oncology (ASCO), May 16–19, Los Angeles, Calif., 17:257a

Setyono Han B, Henkelman MS, Foekens JA, Klijn GM (1987) Direct inhibitory effects of somatostatin (analogues) on the growth of human breast cancer cells. Cancer Res 47:1566–1570

Shiba E, Inoue T, Akazawa K, Takai S (1996) Somatostatin analogue treatment for malignant hypercalcemia associated with advanced breast cancer. Gan To Kagaku Ryoho 23:343–347

Siegel RA, Tolcsvai L, Rudin M (1988) Partial inhibition of the growth of transplanted dunning rat prostate tumors with the long-acting somatostatin analogue Sandostatin (SMS 201-995). Cancer Res 15:16

Smith JP, Solomon TE (1988) Effects of gastrin, proglumide, and somatostatin on growth of human colon cancer. Gastroenterology 95:6

Sperti C, Pasquali C, Catalini S, Cappellazzo F, Bonadimani B, Militello C, Pedrazzoli S (1992) Hormonal treatment of unresectable pancreatic cancer with LHRH analogue (goserelin). Eur J Surg Oncol 18:267–271

Stewart GJ, Connor JL, Lawson JA, Preketes A, King J, Morris DL (1995) Octreotide reduces the kinetic index, proliferating cell nuclear antigen-maximum proliferative index, in patients with colorectal cancer. Cancer 76:572–578

Stewart GJ, Lawson JA, Morris DL (1994) Octreotide inhibits development of hepatic metastases from a human colonic cancer cell line. Br J Surg 81:1332

Stolfi R, Parisi AM, Natoli C, Iacobelli S (1990) Advanced breast cancer: response to somatostatin. Anticancer Res 10:203–204

Sulkowski U, Dinse P, Haus U, Collins W (1997) Regression of a distal bile duct carcinoma after treatment with octreotide for 6 months. Digestion 58:407–409

Suri P, Lipton A, Harvey HA, Wyszynski E, Dixon R, Hamilton RW (1991) Hormonal treatment of pancreatic carcinoma with GNRH and somatostatin analogs. Proc Am Soc Clin Oncol 10:302

Vainas G, Pasaitou V, Galaktidou G, Maris K, Christodoulou K, Constantinidis C, Kortsaris AH (1997) The role of somatostatin analogues in complete antiandrogen treatment in patients with prostatic carcinoma. J Exp Clin Cancer Res 16:1

van Eijck CH, Slooter GD, Hofland LJ, Kort W, Jeekel J, Lamberts SW, Marquet RL (1994) Somatostatin receptor-dependent growth inhibition of liver metastases by octreotide. Br J Surg 9:81

Vennin P, Peyrat JP, Bonneterre J, Louchez MM, Harris AG, Demaille A (1989) Effect of the long-acting somatostatin analogue SMS 201-995 (Sandostatin) in advanced breast cancer. Anticancer Res 9:153–155

Watson SA, Durrant LG, Morris DL (1988) Growth-promoting action of gastrin on human colonic and gastric tumour cells cultured in vitro. Br J Surg 75:4

Weckbecker G, Tolcsvai L, Stolz B, Pollak M, Bruns C (1994) Somatostatin analogue octreotide enhances the antineoplastic effects of tamoxifen and ovariectomy on 7,12-dimethylbenz(alpha)anthracene-induced rat mammary carcinomas. Cancer Res 54:6334–6337

New Molecular Aspects in the Diagnosis and Therapy of Neuroendocrine Tumors of the Gastroenteropancreatic System

U.-F. Pape, M. Höcker, U. Seuß, and B. Wiedenmann

Medizinische Klinik mit Schwerpunkt Hepatologie und Gastroenterologie, Universitätsklinikum Charité, Campus Virchow-Klinikum, Medizinische Fakultät der Humboldt Universität zu Berlin, Augustenburger Platz 1, 13353 Berlin, Germany

Abstract

The nature and biology of neuroendocrine cells and of tumors derived therefrom have been the subject of intense research using cell biological and molecular approaches. Diagnostic procedures for establishing the diagnosis of a neuroendocrine tumor have been improved through the development of new serological markers and imaging procedures. Histopathological diagnosis has been refined by the introduction of a broad spectrum of marker proteins for different subtypes of neuroendocrine neoplasms. The high receptor specificity of somatostatin analogues such as octreotide or lanreotide has made these drugs valuable tools in diagnosis and therapy, and some of the achievements made as well as future directions are reviewed in this article. Another substance in use for therapy of neuroendocrine tumors is interferon-α, whose signal transduction mechanism has been investigated considerably during the past several years. In addition to biotherapy with somatostatin analogues and/or interferon-α, chemotherapy is an accepted strategy in the treatment of advanced neuroendocrine tumor disease derived from the foregut. In this context, streptozotocin has caught some attention due to its somewhat selective toxicity against neuroendocrine tumor cells. Some recent studies on the role of the glucose transporter isoform GLUT2 may provide insight into streptozotocin's action. The multiple endocrine neoplasia type-1 gene has recently been cloned, sequenced and identified as a gene potentially involved in the development of the familial cancer syndrome of multiple endocrine neoplasia type 1 (MEN-1). Mutations of this putative tumor suppressor gene have been described, and the abundance of mutations in MEN-1-related tumors as well as sporadic neuroendocrine tumors at MEN-1 locations have been demonstrated. Whether determination of MEN-1 mutations will be valuable for clinical routine is under investigation.

Recent Results in Cancer Research, Vol. 153
© Springer-Verlag Berlin · Heidelberg 2000

Introduction

Neuroendocrine tumors of the gastroenteropancreatic system have presented a diagnostic and a therapeutic challenge since the first description of the carcinoid syndrome appeared in 1890 (Ranson 1890). Neuroendocrine tumors show a high affinity for silver salts, rendering them argentaffin and/or argyrophil. Argentaffin staining was first introduced by Masson (1914), and it stained neuroendocrine cells in the jejunum and ileum with high specificity. These cells were termed enterochromaffin cells (EC cells), in analogy to the chromaffin cells of the adrenal medulla, to which they were thought to be related. The endocrine nature of EC cells and their scattered distribution throughout the gastrointestinal tract led Feyrter to the concept of the diffuse endocrine system (Feyrter 1938). In 1953, the presence of serotonin (which is thought to be responsible for argentaffinity) was demonstrated in a carcinoid tumor (Lembeck 1953). During the years that followed, the idea of the amine precursor uptake and decarboxylation (APUD) system was developed by Pearse and led to a classification of cells of the diffuse endocrine system by common cytochemical criteria (Pearse 1976). Importantly, these criteria included the abundance of biogenic amines and/or secretory peptide hormones or, under functional aspects, the synthesis and the release of such secretory products, features these cells share with neurons (Langley 1994). In 1968, Grimelius described the argyrophilic reaction as less specific but more sensitive for the staining of neuroendocrine cells (Grimelius 1968). Silver staining methods are still used to detect neuroendocrine cells and neuroendocrine tumors, although their sensitivity for tumor detection varies with location of the tumor (Lloyd 1990). In addition to EC cells, a broad variety of other neuroendocrine cells have been characterized, not only by silver staining but also immunohistochemical methods (Lloyd 1990). Also, ultrastructural subclassifications of neuroendocrine cells were introduced by use of electron microscopy (Langley 1994). In 1995 a revised pathological classification of neuroendocrine tumors was published by Capella et al. (1995), which is based on site of origin, size, invasiveness, and differentiation. For clinical diagnosis, the leading feature is functionality, i.e., the clinical syndromes caused by excess production and secretion of specific biogenic amines and peptide hormones (e.g., the carcinoid syndrome, or hypoglycemia in insulinoma).

Important diagnostic improvements have been made through the development of serological markers and functional provocation tests. Histopathological diagnosis has been improved with the use of a broad spectrum of antibodies in immunohistochemistry recognizing specific marker molecules of neuroendocrine cells. The introduction of somatostatin analogues such as octreotide and lanreotide was a highly specific diagnostic and therapeutic approach when it started in the 1980s, and it has given rise to further developments in specific therapy. These include both diagnosis using somatostatin receptor scintigraphy and biotherapy with somatostatin analogues and also interferon-α. A tumor-specific approach employs streptozotocin as part of a chemotherapeutic regimen for neuroendocrine tumors located in the foregut, even though the precise cellular mechanisms are not yet understood. This article also reviews recent developments with respect to the molecular diagnosis of neuroendocrine tumors, including descriptions of mutations of the multiple endocrine neoplasia type-1 (MEN-1) gene mutations.

Laboratory Studies

The most widely used marker for neuroendocrine tumors is chromogranin A, an integral matrix protein of large dense-core vesicles (LDCV) of neuroendocrine cells. Chromogranin A is a 48-kD member of the granin family of proteins which assists in vesicle stabilization, pro-hormone processing, and regulation of secretion. Serum chromogranin A has been shown to be an excellent general marker for neuroendocrine neoplasia, although no correlation with functionality has been established (Deftos et al. 1988; Wiedenmann and Huttner 1989; Schürmann et al. 1992). Additionally, chromogranin A appears to be superior with respect to sensitivity and/or specificity when compared with other neuroendocrine tumor markers, such as neuron-specific enolase (NSE) (Nobels et al. 1997). Interestingly, some subtypes of neuroendocrine tumors do not stain for, and probably also do not secrete, chromogranin A and thus could escape routine laboratory screening for neuroendocrine neoplasia (Fahrenkamp et al. 1995). On the other hand, hypergastrinemia in chronic atrophic gastritis or treatment with proton-pump inhibitors (PPIs) may lead to elevated serum chromogranin A levels (Borch et al. 1997; Simon et al. 1995). Thus, chromogranin A should not be the only tumor marker determined in suspected neuroendocrine tumor disease, because both false-negative and false-positive results can be misleading.

Therefore, additional diagnostic information should be obtained from determination of specific hormones or peptides (Table 1) in patient serum. Furthermore, provocation tests, such as the secretin test

Table 1. Diagnostic markers and tests for gastroenteropancreatic neuroendocrine neoplasms (*NSE* neuron-specific enolase)

Neuroendocrine tumor	Serum marker/provocation test	Immunostaining
General	Chromogranin A	Chromogranin A Synaptophysin NSE[a]
Carcinoid	Serotonin[b], 5-HIAA (24-h urinary sample)	Serotonin
Gastrinoma	Gastrin/secretin test	Gastrin
Insulinoma	Insulin, C-peptide/24-h fasting test	Insulin
Glucagonoma	Glucagon	Glucagon
VIPoma	Vasoactive intestinal polypeptide (VIP)	VIP
Somatostatinoma	Somatostatin	Somatostatin
PPoma	Pancreatic polypeptide (PP)	PP
ACTHoma	Adrenocorticotropic hormone (ACTH)	ACTH
ECLoma	Gastrin (not in sporadic or MEN-1-associated cases)	VMAT-2 (?)

[a] No longer a standard. [b] Not established as standard.

for establishing the diagnosis of a gastrinoma, have been in use. Patients with Zollinger-Ellison syndrome caused by a gastrinoma demonstrate a characteristic increase of serum gastrin levels on i.v. administration of secretin. However, patients with relapsing peptic ulcer disease often have been started on PPIs such as omeprazole without a Zollinger-Ellison syndrome first being ruled out. Such patients also have elevated basal serum gastrin levels, but they do not demonstrate the diagnostic increase of more than 200 pg/ml of serum gastrin in response to i.v. administration of secretin, making the diagnosis of gastrinoma unlikely (Meko and Norton 1995).

Other stimulatory tests for detection of nonfunctional neuroendocrine tumors, such as the pentagastrin test, which has already been useful in the diagnosis of medullary thyroid carcinoma, or the calcium infusion test, have been investigated (Ahlman et al. 1996). However, routine clinical use of provocation tests other than the secretin test cannot be recommended currently, because the results from their clinical application have been unreliable and have not improved the diagnostic process of neuroendocrine tumors. It is important to keep in mind that the administration of antisecretory drugs (i.e., somatostatin analogues or PPIs) should be stopped, if possible, before such tests are performed. However, other strategies such as somatostatin receptor imaging or endoscopic ultrasonography may be more sensitive in detecting subclinical disease (Zimmer et al. 1994, 1995). Although imaging techniques provide evidence about tumor localization, stimulatory tests give early information on functionality of a suspected or proven neuroendocrine tumor.

Immunohistochemical Diagnosis

Major progress in the histological diagnosis of neuroendocrine neoplasias was made in the late 1980s with the introduction of immunohistochemical staining against synaptophysin and chromogranin A (Wiedenmann et al. 1986; Wiedenmann et al. 1988; Wiedenmann and Huttner 1989). In contrast to chromogranin A, synaptophysin is a membrane component of the small synaptic vesicles (SSV) of neuronal and neuroendocrine cells. SSVs contain nonpeptidergic transmitters such as amino acid transmitters, amines, gamma amino butyric acid (GABA), and acetylcholine. Synaptophysin participates in the docking and fusion process during exocytosis in concert with other molecules such as the synaptobrevins or syntaxins. Specific expression of major proteins characteristic for regulated exocytosis by the synaptosomal-associated protein receptor (SNARE) complex has been demonstrated (Ahnert-Hilger et al. 1996). Expression of cell type-specific isoforms of synaptosomal-associated protein SNAP 25, the syntaxins, and synaptobrevin in both neuroendocrine pancreatic tumors and human pancreatic islets different from SNARE proteins present in normal exocrine pancreatic tissue has been observed, and thus similarity between neuronal cells and pancreatic neuroendocrine cells with respect to SNARE protein expression and exocytotic function has been shown (Ahnert-Hilger et al. 1993; Ahnert-Hilger et al. 1996). However, chromogranin A and synaptophysin are still the most widely used defining immunohistochemical markers for neuroendocrine tumors (Capella et al. 1995).

Accumulation of monoamines such as histamine in secretory vesicles of neuroendocrine cells is mediated by specific vesicular monoamine transporters (VMAT) (Nirenberg et al. 1995). A new isoform of VMATs which localizes to the membrane of secretory vesicles such as SSV has recently been cloned and localized to neuronal and neuroendocrine cells (Erickson et al. 1996). Interestingly, the VMAT-2 isoform shows a selective expression in the enterochromaffin-like (ECL) cells of the gastric mucosa, and a role for histamine transport has been suggested (Dimaline and Struthers 1996; Zhao et al. 1997). It remains to be seen whether VMAT-2 staining will allow a subclassification of gastric synaptophysin/chromogranin A-positive cells. Discrimination between benign ECL-cell tumors and gastric neuroendocrine neoplasms may be an attractive application for VMAT-2 staining in the future.

A more detailed characterization of neuroendocrine neoplasias which stain positive for the general markers (i.e., synaptophysin and/or chromogranin A) can be obtained by staining for specific hormone or peptide products (Table 1). Many of the neuroendocrine tumors which stain positive for biogenic amines or peptide hormones remain clinically silent and have to be classified as nonfunctional neoplasms (Moertel 1987). Immunohistochemical staining for the nuclear Ki67-antigen has become a widely used pathological method for evaluating proliferating cells in a certain tumor (Gerdes et al. 1983; Bruno et al. 1991). Staining of neuroendocrine neoplasms for the Ki67-antigen provides an estimate about the proliferating cell fraction within a single tumor and helps in judging the biological behavior of the tumor (Öberg 1994). A similar approach has been the application of proliferating cell nuclear antigen (PCNA) and determination of differences in immunoreactivity for PCNA between benign and malignant neuroendocrine tumors (Wang et al. 1997). However, the use of Ki67 or PCNA is not yet considered a standard procedure (Capella et al. 1995), because their precise value for assessing the malignant potential of a neuroendocrine neoplasm has not yet been determined.

Somatostatin Receptors and Somatostatin Analogues – Diagnosis and Therapy with Molecular Specificity

Major progress was made in the diagnosis of neuroendocrine tumors with the introduction of somatostatin receptor scintigraphy, which has become the standard first-line method for localizing neuroendocrine neoplasms (Krenning et al. 1994; Zimmer et al. 1994; Wiedenmann et al. 1994). Two innovations were necessary for such progress, one being the pharmacological and molecular characterization of somatostatin receptors (for review see: Reubi 1997; Tang et al. 1997). The other was the successful development of stable somatostatin analogues such as octreotide and lanreotide. Neuroendocrine tumors express receptors for both human somatostatins (somatostatin-14 and -28). The somatostatin analogues octreotide and lanreotide are also able to bind to these receptors, although with differing affinities (Reubi 1997; Schaer et al. 1997; Tang et al. 1997). To date, five human somatostatin receptor subtypes (hSSTR 1-5) have been identified. In neuroendocrine gastroenteropancreatic tumors hSSTR subtypes 1, 2, and 5 seem to be preferentially expressed, whereas a high abundance of the hSSTR subtype 3 is found in brain and pituitary tumors (Schaer et al. 1997; Jonas et al. 1995). This is of importance for the clinical application of octreotide and lanreotide, which bind with high affinity only to the hSSTR subtypes 2 and 5, as opposed to naturally occurring ligands, which bind to all receptor subtypes with relatively high although differing affinities (Reisine and Bell 1995). Preferential expression of hSSTR subtype 2 in neuroendocrine tumors and the high affinity of octreotide and lanreotide for hSSTR subtype 2 complement each other for tumor detection and therapeutic purposes. On the other hand, some neuroendocrine tumors such as insulinomas display low expression of hSSTR subtype 2, which thus may be harder to detect with [111]indium-labeled octreotide (Wiedenmann et al. 1994; John et al. 1996). For these neoplasms additional diagnostic procedures such as endoscopic ultrasonography are more sensitive (Zimmer et al. 1994).

Radioactively labeled octreotide has also been injected preoperatively, followed by intraoperative tracing with a scintillation probe to detect hSSTR-expressing tumor tissue (Ahlman et al. 1994). It may soon be possible to localize preoperatively unknown tumors intraoperatively and then resect them. Although this method is still hampered by technical problems, it may benefit patients with primary tumors of unknown localization by allowing a more accurate assessment of metastatic disease and more thorough resection.

Due to their inhibitory action on the secretion and proliferation of neuroendocrine tumor cells, the clinical use of somatostatin analogues is widely accepted. The most important indications to date are the various hypersecretion syndromes of neuroendocrine tumors, ranging from the classical carcinoid syndrome to the life-threatening malignant carcinoid crisis (for which somatostatin analogues present the only really effective therapy; Moertel 1987). Recently, depot formulations have become available, allowing a more convenient intramuscular injection once every 2 or even 4 weeks, but s.c. injection three times daily is still the standard method of administration (Scherübl et al. 1994; Faiss et al. 1996a).

Several mechanisms have been postulated to underlie the antiproliferative effect of somatostatin. Influences on a broad variety of intracellular signal transduction pathways such as inhibition of the MAP kinase pathway, inhibition of the transcription factor complex activator protein-1 (AP-1), or activation of phosphoprotein phosphatases have been demonstrated in various cell culture models, but their precise role in neuroendocrine tumors is not yet understood (Ren et al. 1992; Todisco et al. 1995; Cordelier et al. 1997; Bousquet et al. 1998). Also suggested is an antiproliferative effect of somatostatin and its analogues through inhibition of auto- and paracrine stimulation of tumor growth by secretory products such as insulin, epidermal growth factor, or growth hormone (Reisine and Bell 1995). Clinical relevance of somatostatin-mediated antiproliferative effects was shown, at least in part, in a German multicenter trial which demonstrated octreotide-mediated inhibition of tumor growth of previously progressive disease, resulting in a stable disease situation (Arnold et al. 1996). However, no partial or complete remission as determined by imaging studies was observed. In contrast, from clinical trials using ultra-high-dose regimens of the somatostatin analogue lanreotide, partial remissions and even one complete remission as determined by imaging studies have been reported (Faiss et al. 1996b; Eriksson et al. 1997). Again, stabilization of previously progressive disease was the major clinical and morphological effect in 43–70% of the patients in these studies. In both studies, however, up to 43% of the patients still showed progressive disease (Faiss et al. 1996b; Eriksson et al. 1997). Thus, it is not entirely clear to what extent octreotide-mediated inhibition of cell proliferation clinically contributes to the inhibition of progressive tumor disease.

A future perspective is the use of somatostatin analogues as highly specific carrier molecules for cytotoxic radioisotopes such as ^{111}In or ^{90}Y. The radioactive substance can be delivered to malignant tumor cells via endocytosis of receptor-bound somatostatin analogues. hSSTRs are classical seven-transmembrane-spanning-domain, G-protein-coupled receptors, which become internalized once the ligand is bound. The concept is to label a somatostatin analogue with high specificity for a particular hSSTR (e.g., hSSTR subtype 2) with an α- or β-emitting radioisotope such as ^{90}Y and thus achieve a high specificity for tumor-directed radiotherapy (Lamberts et al. 1994; McCarthy et al. 1998; Otte et al. 1998). Interestingly, a similar approach using vasoactive intestinal polypeptide (VIP) as a ligand molecule has been evaluated for imaging neuroendocrine tumors and various adenocarcinomas (Virgolini et al. 1994). These studies demonstrated visualization of both tumor types. However, VIP-receptor imaging does not appear to be as sensitive and specific as somatostatin receptor scintigraphy for neuroendocrine tumors (Virgolini et al. 1994).

Interferon-α – Partner in Biotherapy

Interferon-α has been used as a therapeutic agent for neuroendocrine tumors alone or in combination with either somatostatin analogues or chemotherapy (Öberg et al. 1994; Faiss et al. 1996a). Its action on neuroendocrine tumors includes antiproliferative effects, induction of apoptosis, differentiation, and immunomodulation (Öberg et al. 1994). The cellular mechanisms of interferon-α action have been elucidated during the past few years: Activation of interferon-α receptors results in receptor dimerization and subsequent stimulation of associated kinases of the janus kinase family (JAK) through tyrosine phosphorylation. JAKs, in turn, phosphorylate STAT (signal transducers and activators of transcription) molecules, which dimerize and translocate into the nucleus, where they act as transcription factors (Ransohoff 1998; Haque and Williams 1998). A broad variety of probably more than 100 genes can be regulated through interferon-α action, and in neuroendocrine tumors the 2'-5'-A-synthetase gene or the apoptosis genes bcl-2 and bax have been identified as interferon target genes (Öberg et al. 1994; Imam et al. 1997). However, the exact molecular nature of the effects interferon-α has on neuroendocrine tumors, resulting in inhibition of proliferation, has to be elucidated.

Treatment of neuroendocrine tumors with interferon-α has resulted in a morphological response of the tumor, as determined by an at least 50% reduction in tumor size on imaging studies in up to only 20% of patients treated with interferon-α (Öberg et al. 1994). This has been partially explained by an induction of fibrosis in liver metastasis, the most frequently used reference in the follow-up of neuroendocrine tumors. This fibrotic process was not detectable by conventional imaging studies such as CT scans and ultrasonography (Öberg et al. 1994). Important limiting factors in the treatment of patients with interferon-α are adverse reactions such as flu-like symptoms, fatigue, low-grade weight loss, mental depression, elevated liver enzymes, or autoimmune disease (Öberg et al. 1994). The activation of cytosolic phospholipase A_2 through activation of the interferon-α receptor has been observed. Although it is not known whether phospholipase A_2 activation provides some of the antitumor effects of interferon-α, it has been speculated that it might contribute to the clinical side effects of interferon-α therapy (Haque and Williams 1998).

It is important for the clinical application of interferon-α that antibodies against recombinant interferon-α may occur. These antibodies can bind to most of the recombinant interferons in clinical use, but they neutralize the actions of interferon-α in only a small percentage of patients (Bordens et al. 1997). However, in such patients a change to human leukocyte interferon may restore interferon-α effects (Öberg et al. 1994).

Chemotherapy: Streptozotocin as a Tumor-specific Drug?

Chemotherapy was the major treatment for neuroendocrine tumors before biotherapy was introduced in the 1980s, and it still is for malignant, more rapidly growing neuroendocrine tumors. One of the most common regimens, especially for foregut tumors, is the combination of streptozotocin with 5-fluorouracil (Moertel 1987; Eriksson et al. 1990; Arnold and Frank 1995). Streptozotocin and the related compound chlorozotocin are glucose molecules with a nitrosourea substitute in the C_2 position. The nitrosourea component is most likely the actual toxic part of the molecule (Calabresi and Chabner 1991).

Little is known about the cellular mechanism by which streptozotocin exerts its toxic effects, but it has been shown that streptozotocin uses the glucose transporter GLUT2 to enter pancreatic β-cells (Schnedl et al. 1994). GLUT2 is the glucose-dependent isoform of the glucose transporter molecule and is preferentially expressed in pancreatic β-cells. The affinity of this transporter molecule to streptozotocin and its preferential expression in pancreatic islets provides the potential basis for the cell-specific action of streptozotocin. However, it is still unclear how streptozotocin exerts its cellular toxicity. Interestingly, multiple low-dose injections of streptozotocin into mice resulted in a decrease of GLUT2 mRNA and protein, possibly providing evidence for a protective mechanism of β-cells against streptozotocin-related cytotoxic effects (Wang et al. 1998). Another important mechanism that might contribute to streptozotocin-related toxicity is a T-cell-mediated immune reaction which follows streptozotocin administration. Insulinitis, with subsequent islet-cell destruction and diabetes mellitus, has been shown as a consequence of a macrophage infiltrate which follows streptozotocin-induced neoantigen expression on the β-cells (Fraser et al. 1997). However, it is not known whether similar processes occur in neuroendocrine foregut tumors treated with streptozotocin.

Genetic Diagnosis of Neuroendocrine Neoplasms

Multiple endocrine neoplasia type 1 (MEN-1) is a familial cancer syndrome inherited in an autosomal-dominant pattern in affected families. Patients demonstrate in varying combinations tumors of the parathyroid, the anterior pituitary, and pancreatic islets. Although less common, other foregut neuroendocrine tumors may also be associated with this syndrome. In 1997 the nucleic acid sequence of a putative tumor-suppressor gene associated with MEN-1 was cloned and localized to chromosome 11q13. The gene product was termed menin, and 12 different mutations of the MEN-1 gene were demonstrated in 15 unrelated MEN-1 patients (Chandrasehkharappa et al. 1997). In a series of further publications, this group demonstrated mutations in the MEN-1 gene in sporadic pituitary tumors, parathyroid tumors, carcinoid lung tumors, and gastrinomas, as well as in insulinomas. However, at 17–36%, the incidence of mutations was considerably lower in patients with sporadic tumors than the 80% mutation rate in MEN-1 patients (Zhuang et al. 1997a; Heppner et al. 1997; Debelenko et al. 1997; Zhuang et al. 1997b). In sporadic gastroenteropancreatic neuroendocrine tumors, MEN-1 gene mutations seem to be restricted to foregut neoplasms (Toliat et al. 1997). Hessman et al. (1998) also reported MEN-1 gene mutations in nonfamilial, malignant, endocrine pancreatic tumors and described various mutations which could potentially lead to impaired menin function. As has been shown for other tumor suppressor genes, mutations in the MEN-1 gene seem to play a major role in tumorigenesis only when loss of heterozygosity occurs.

Recently, a first description of a possible functional role for menin was published by Guru et al. (1998), who describe a primarily nuclear localization of the menin protein. Although menin lacks the classical nuclear localization sequences (NLS), two potential NLS were detected through deletion constructs of menin (Guru et al. 1998). Interestingly, 39 of the meanwhile 43 known mutations of the MEN-1 gene result in a loss of both NLS, thus leading to severely, if not totally, impaired translocation of menin from the cytoplasm into the nucleus. However, the functional relevance of a cytosolic versus a nuclear localization of menin is not yet known, nor is its actual function.

With the role of MEN-1 gene mutations becoming clearer, the gene's importance for tumorigenesis and eventual therapeutic strategies may become manifest. This will be of particular interest to MEN-1 patients, since their hereditary condition and precancerous state may be diagnosed early and thus be accessible to cancer prevention strategies.

Conclusions

The biology of neuroendocrine cells has been investigated intensively, and some of the most important results with actual or possible diagnostic or therapeutic impact have been mentioned here. However, it should be noted that a definitive cure of a gastroenteropancreatic neuroendocrine tumor is still possible exclusively through surgery, and that careful preoperative diagnosis is a requirement for choosing the right surgical approach when one is operating with curative intent (Wiedenmann et al. 1998). Somatostatin receptor scintigraphy is thus central to both surgical and conservative therapy. Where palliation is concerned, particularly biotherapy with somatostatin analogues and interferon-α has improved the clinical outcome of patients with neuroendocrine tumors. Further efforts to improve diagnosis and therapy are still required. Receptor-targeted radiotherapy could be a promising aspect in this area. Improvement of chemotherapeutic regimens for neuroendocrine tumors with potentially "tumor-specific" substances such as streptozotocin also deserves further attention. More cell-specific derivatives of streptozotocin could provide a therapeutic perspective for future research. We have just begun to take genetic approaches to the diagnosis of neuroendocrine tumors. In the near future we can expect to see diagnostic benefit from genetic screening for menin mutations. Some encouraging progress has been made over the past decade in the diagnosis and treatment of neuroendocrine neoplasms, but many questions remain to be solved, and continued research to improve current strategies is necessary.

References

Ahlman H, Tisell LE, Wängberg B, Nilsson O, Forssell-Aronsson E, Fjälling M (1994) Somatostatin receptor imaging in patients with neuroendocrine tumors: preoperative and postoperative scintigraphy and intraoperative use of a scintillation detector. Semin Oncol 21 [Suppl 13]:21–28

Ahlman H, Nilsson O, Wängberg B, Dahlström A (1996) Neuroendocrine insights from the laboratory to the clinic. Am J Surg 172:61–67

Ahnert-Hilger G, Grube K, Kvols L, Lee I, Mönch E, Riecken EO, Schmitt L, Wiedenmann B (1993) Gastroenteropancreatic neuroendocrine tumours contain a common set of synaptic vesicle proteins and amino acid neurotransmitters. Eur J Cancer 29A:1982–1984

Ahnert-Hilger G, Stadtbäumer A, Strübing C, Scherübl H, Schultz G, Riecken EO, Wiedenmann B (1996) γ-Aminobutyric acid secretion from pancreatic neuroendocrine cells. Gastroenterology 110:1595–1604

Arnold R, Frank M (1995) Systemic chemotherapy for endocrine tumors of the pancreas: recent advances. Front Gastrointest Res 23:431–438

Arnold R, Trautmann ME, Creutzfeld W, Benning R, Benning M, Neuhaus C, Jürgensen R, Stein K, Schäfer H, Bruns C, Dennler HJ (1996) Somatostatin analogue octreotide and inhibition of tumor growth in metastatic endocrine gastroenteropancreatic tumours. Gut 38:430–438

Bellmann K, Wenz A, Radons J, Burkart V, Kleemann R, Kolb H (1995) Heat shock induces resistance in rat pancreatic islet cells against nitric oxide, oxygen radicals and streptozotocin toxicity in vitro. J Clin Invest 95:2840–2845

Borch K, Stridsberg M, Burman P, Rehfeld JF (1997) Basal chromogranin A and gastrin concentrations in circulation correlate to endocrine cell proliferation in type-A gastritis. Scand J Gastroenterol 32:198–202

Bordens R, Grossberg SE, Trotta PP, Nagabhushan TL (1997) Molecular and biologic characterization of recombinant interferon-α_{2b}. Semin Oncol 24 [Suppl 9]:S9-41–S9-51

Bouquet C, Delesque N, Lopez F, Saint-Laurent N, Estève JP, Bedecs K, Buscail L, Vaysse N, Susini C (1998) sst2 Somatostatin receptor mediates negative regulation of insulin receptor signaling through the tyrosine phosphatase SHP-1. J Biol Chem 273:7099–7106

Bruno S, Crissman HA, Bauer KD, Darzynkiewicz Z (1991) Changes in cell nuclei during S phase: positive chromatin condensation and altered expression of the proliferation-associated nuclear proteins Ki67, cyclin (PCNA), p105, and p34. Exp Cell Res 196:99–106

Calabresi P, Chabner BA (1991) Antineoplastic agents. In: Goodman Gilman A, Rall TW, Nies AS, Taylor P (eds) Goodman & Gilman's the pharmacological basis of therapeutics, chap 52. Pergamon, New York, pp 1209–1263

Capella C, Heitz PU, Höfler H, Solcia E, Klöppel G (1995) Revised classification of neuroendocrine tumors of the lung, pancreas and gut. Virchows Arch 425:547–560

Chandrasekharappa SC, Guru SC, Manickam P, Olufemi SE, Collins FS, Emmert-Buck MR, Debelenko LV, Zhuang Z, Lubensky IA, Liotta LA, Crabtree JS, Wang Y, Roe BA, Weisemann J, Boguski MS, Agarwal SK, Kester MB, Kim YS, Heppner C, Dong Q, Spiegel AM, Burns AL, Marx SJ (1997) Positional cloning of the gene for multiple endocrine neoplasia-type 1. Science 276:404–407

Cordelier P, Estève JP, Bousquet C, Delesque N, O'Carroll AM, Schally AV, Vaysse N, Susini C, Buscail L (1997) Characterization of the antiproliferative signal mediated by the somatostatin receptor subtype sst 5. Proc Natl Acad Sci USA 94:93439348

Debelenko LV, Brambilla E, Agarwal SK, Swalwell JI, Kester MB, Lubensky IA, Zhuang Z, Guru SC, Manickam P, Olufemi SE, Chandrasekharappa SC, Crabtree JS, Kim YS, Heppner C, Burns AL, Spiegel AM, Marx SJ, Liotta LA, Collins FS, Travis WD, Emmert-Buck MR (1997) Identification of MEN1 gene mutations in sporadic carcinoid tumors of the lung. Hum Mol Genet 6:2285–2290

Deftos LJ, Linnoila RI, Carney DN, Burton DW, Leong SS, O'Connor DT, Murray SS, Gazdar AF (1988) Demonstration of chromogranin A in human neuroendocrine cell lines by immunohistology and immunoassay. Cancer 62:92–97

Dimaline R, Struthers J (1996) Expression and regulation of a vesicular monoamine transporter in rat stomach: a putative histamine transporter. J Physiol (Lond) 490:249–256

Eriksson B, Skogseid B, Lundqvist G, Wide L, Wilander E, Öberg K (1990) Medical treatment and long-term survival in a prospective study of 84 patients with endocrine pancreatic tumors. Cancer 65:1883–1890

Eriksson B, Renstrup J, Imam H, Öberg K (1997) High-dose treatment with lanreotide of patients with advanced neuroendocrine gastrointestinal tumors: clinical and biological effects. Ann Oncol 8:1041–1044

Erickson JD, Schafer MK, Bonner TI, Eiden LE, Weihe E (1996) Distinct pharmacological properties and distribution in neurons and endocrine cells of two isoforms of the human vesicular monoamine transporter. Proc Natl Acad Sci USA 93:5166–5171

Fahrenkamp AG, Wibbeke C, Winde G, Ofner D, Böcker W, Fischer-Colbrie R, Schmid KW (1995) Immunohistochemical distribution of chromogranins A and B and secretogranin II in neuroendocrine tumours of the gastrointestinal tract. Virchows Arch 426:361–367

Faiss S, Scherübl H, Riecken EO, Wiedenmann B (1996a) Drug therapy in metastatic neuroendocrine tumors of the gastroenteropancreatic system. Recent Results Cancer Res 142:193–207

Faiss S, Scherübl H, Riecken EO, Wiedenmann B (1996b) Interferon-α versus somatostatin or the combination of both in metastatic neuroendocrine gut and pancreatic tumours. Digestion 57 [Suppl 1]:84–85

Feyrter F (1938) Über diffuse endokrine epitheliale Organe. Zbl Inn Med 59:545

Fraser RB, Rowden G, Colp P, Wright JR (1997) Immunophenotyping of insulitis in control and essential fatty acid-deficient mice treated with multiple low-dose streptozotocin. Diabetologia 40:1263–1268

Gerdes J, Schwab U, Lemke H, Stein H (1983) Production of a mouse monoclonal antibody reactive with a human nuclear antigen associated with cell proliferation. Int J Cancer 31:13–20

Grimelius L (1968) A silver nitrate stain for a_2 cells in human pancreatic islets. Acta Soc Med Upsal 73:243–270

Guru SC, Goldsmith PK, Burns AL, Marx SJ, Spiegel AM, Collins FS, Chandrasekharappa SC (1998) Menin, the product of the MEN1 gene, is a nuclear protein. Proc Natl Acad Sci USA 95:1630–1634

Haque SJ, Williams BRG (1998) Signal transduction in the interferon system. Semin Oncol 25 [Suppl 1]:14–22

Heppner C, Kester MB, Agarwal SK, Debelenko LV, Emmert-Buck MR, Guru SC, Manickam P, Olufemi SE, Skarulis MC, Doppman JL, Alexander RH, Kim YS, Saggar SK, Lubensky IA, Zhuang Z, Liotta LA, Chandrasekharappa SC, Collins FS, Spiegel AM, Burns AL, Marx SJ (1997) Somatic mutation of the MEN1 gene in parathyroid tumors. Nature Genet 16:375–378

Hessman O, Lindberg D, Skogseid B, Carling T, Hellman P, Rastad J, Akerström G, Westin G (1998) Mutation of the multiple endocrine neoplasia type 1 gene in nonfamilial malignant tumors of the endocrine pancreas. Cancer Res 58:377–379

Imam H, Gobl A, Eriksson B, Öberg K (1997) Interferon-alpha induces bcl-2 proto-oncogene in patients with neuroendocrine gut tumor responding to its antitumor action. Anticancer Res 17:4659–4665

John M, Meyerhof W, Richter D, Waser B, Schaer JC, Scherübl H, Boese-Landgraf J, Neuhaus P, Ziske C, Mölling K, Riecken EO, Reubi JC, Wiedenmann B (1996) Positive somatostatin receptor scintigraphy correlates with the presence of somatostatin receptor subtype 2 and 5. Gut 38:33–39

Jonas S, John M, Boese-Landgraf J, Häring R, Prevost G, Thomas F, Rosewicz S, Riecken EO, Wiedenmann B, Neuhaus P (1995) Somatostatin receptor subtypes in neuroendocrine tumor cell lines and tumor tissues. Langenbecks Arch Chir 380:90–95

Krenning EP, Kwekkeboom DJ, Oel HY, DeJong RJB, Dop FJ, Reubi JC, Lamberts SWJ (1994) Somatostatin-receptor scintigraphy in gastroenteropancreatic tumors. Ann NY Acad Sci 733:416–424

Lamberts SWJ, Reubi JC, Krenning EP (1994) The role of somatostatin analogues in the control of tumor growth. Semin Oncol 21 [Suppl 13]:61–64

Langley K (1994) The neuroendocrine concept today. Ann NY Acad Sci 733:1–17

Lembeck F (1953) 5-Hydroxytryptamine in a carcinoid tumor. Nature 172:910

Lloyd RV (1990) Endocrine pathology. Springer, Berlin Heidelberg New York

Masson P (1914) La glande endocrine de l'intestine chez l'homme. CR Acad Sci 158:52–61

McCarthy KE, Woltering EA, Espenan GD, Cronin M, Maloney TJ, Anthony LB (1998) In situ radiotherapy with ^{111}In-pentetreotide: initial observations and future directions. Cancer J Sci Am 4:94–102

Meko JB, Norton JA (1995) Management of patients with Zollinger-Ellison syndrome. Ann Rev Med 46:395–411

Moertel CG (1987) An odyssey in the land of small tumors. J Clin Oncol 5:1503–1522

Nirenberg MJ, Liu Y, Peter D, Edwards RH, Pickel VM (1995) The vesicular monoamine transporter 2 is present in small synaptic vesicles and preferentially localizes to large dense core vesicles in rat solitary tract nuclei. Proc Natl Acad Sci USA 92:8773–8777

Nobels FR, Kwekkeboom DJ, Coopmans W, Schoenmakers CH, Lindemans J, DeHerder WW, Krenning EP, Bouillon R, Lamberts SW (1997) Chromogranin A as serum marker for neuroendocrine neoplasia: comparison with neuron-specific enolase and the alpha-subunit of glycoprotein hormones. J Clin Endocrinol Metab 82:2622–2628

Nwokolo CU, Debnam ES, Booth JD, Sim R, Sankey EA, Dhillon AP, Pounder RE (1992) Neuroendocrine changes in rat stomach during experimental diabetes mellitus. Dig Dis Sci 37:751–756

Öberg K (1994) Expression of growth factors and their receptors in neuroendocrine gut and pancreas tumors, and prognostic factors for survival. Ann NY Acad Sci 733:46–55

Öberg K, Eriksson B, Janson ET (1994) The clinical use of interferons in the management of neuroendocrine gastroenteropancreatic tumors. Ann NY Acad Sci 733:471–478

Otte A, Mueller-Brand J, Dellas S, Nitzsche EU, Herrmann R, Maecke HR (1998) Yttrium-90-labelled somatostatin analogue for cancer treatment. Lancet 351:417–418

Pearse AGE (1976) Peptides in brain and intestine. Nature 262:92–94

Ransohoff RM (1998) Cellular responses to interferons and other cytokines: the JAK-STAT paradigm. N Engl J Med 338:616–618

Ranson WB (1890) A case of primary carcinoma of the ileum. Lancet 2:1020

Reisine T, Bell GI (1995) Molecular biology of somatostatin receptors. Endocr Rev 16:427–442

Ren SG, Ezzat S, Melmed S, Braunstein GD (1992) Somatostatin analogue induces insulin-like growth factor binding protein-1 (IGFBP-1) expression in human hepatoma cells. Endocrinology 131:2479–2481

Reubi JC (1997) Relevance of somatostatin receptors and other peptide receptors in pathology. Endocrine Pathol 8:11–20

Schaer JC, Waser B, Mengod G, Reubi JC (1997) Somatostatin receptor subtypes sst_1, sst_2, sst_3, and sst_5 expression in human pituitary, gastroentero-pancreatic and mammary tumors: comparison of mRNA analysis with receptor autoradiography. Int J Cancer 70:530–537

Scherübl H, Wiedenmann B, Riecken EO, Thomas F, Böhme E, Räth U (1994) Treatment of the carcinoid syndrome with a depot formulation of the somatostatin analogue lanreotide. Eur J Cancer 6:1590–1591

Schnedl WJ, Ferber S, Johnson JH, Newgard CB (1994) STZ transport and cytotoxicity. Specific enhancement in GLUT2-expressing cells. Diabetes 43:1326–1333

Schürmann G, Raeth U, Wiedenmann B, Buhr H, Herfarth C (1992) Serum chromogranin A in the diagnosis and follow-up of neuroendocrine tumors of the gastroenteropancreatic tract. World J Surg 16:697–702

Simon B, Eissele R, Czornik M, Swarovsky B, Arnold R (1995) Effect of gastrin receptor blockade on gastrin and histidine decarboxylase gene expression in rats during achlohydria. Scand J Gastroenterol 30:503–510

Tang C, Biemond I, Lamers CB (1997) Expression of peptide receptors in human endocrine tumours of the pancreas. Gut 40:267–271

Todisco A, Seva C, Takeuchi Y, Dickinson CJ, Yamada T (1995) Somatostatin inhibits AP-1 function via multiple protein phosphatases. Am J Physiol 269:G160–166

Toliat MR, Berger W, Ropers HH, Neuhaus P, Wiedenmann B (1997) Mutations in the MEN-I gene in sporadic neuroendocrine tumours of the gastroenteropancreatic system. Lancet 350:1223

Virgolini I, Raderer M, Kurtaran A, Angelberger P, Banyai S, Yang Q, Li S, Banyai M, Pidlich J, Niederle B, Scheithauer W, Valent P (1994) Vasoactive intestinal peptide-receptor imaging for the localization of intestinal adenocarcinomas and endocrine tumors. N Engl J Med 331:1116–1121

Wang Z, Gleichmann H (1998) GLUT2 in pancreatic islets: crucial target molecule in diabetes induced with multiple low doses of streptozotocin in mice. Diabetes 47:50–56

Wang DG, Johnston CF, Buchanan KD (1997) Oncogene expression in gastroenteropancreatic neuroendocrine tumors. Cancer 80:668–675

Wiedenmann B, Huttner WB (1989) Synaptophysin and chromogranins/secretogranins: widespread constituents of distinct types of neuroendocrine vesicles and new tools in tumor diagnosis. Virchows Arch 58:95–121

Wiedenmann B, Franke WW, Kuhn C, Moll R, Gould V (1986) Synaptophysin: a marker protein for neuroendocrine cells and neoplasms. Proc Natl Acad Sci USA 83:3500–3504

Wiedenmann B, Waldherr R, Buhr H, Hille A, Rosa P, Huttner WB (1988) Identification of gastroenteropancreatic neuroendocrine cells in normal and neoplastic human tissue with antibodies against synaptophysin, chromogranin A, secretogranin I (chromogranin B), and secretogranin II. Gastroenterology 95:1364–1374

Wiedenmann B, Bäder HM, Scherübl H, Fett U, Zimmer T, Hamm B, Koppenhagen K, Riecken EO (1994) Gastroenteropancreatic tumor imaging with somatostatin receptor scintigraphy. Semin Oncol 21 [Suppl 13]:29–32

Wiedenmann B, Jensen RT, Mignon M, Modlin CI, Skogseid B, Doherty G, Öberg K (1998) Preoperative diagnosis and surgical management of neuroendocrine gastroenteropancreatic tumors: general recommendations by a consensus workshop. World J Surg 22:309–318

Zhao CM, Jacobsson G, Chen D, Hakanson R, Meister B (1997) Exocytotic proteins in enterochromaffin-like (ECL) cells of the rat stomach. Cell Tissue Res 290:539–551

Zhuang Z, Ezzat SZ, Vortmeyer AO, Weil R, Oldfield EH, Park WS, Pack S, Huang S, Agarwal SK, Guru SC, Manickam P, Debelenko LV, Kester MB, Olufemi SE, Heppner C, Crabtree JS, Burns AL, Spiegel AM, Marx SJ, Chandrasekharappa SC, Collins FS, Emmert-Buck MR, Liotta LA, Asa SL, Lubensky IA (1997a) Mutations of the MEN1 tumor suppressor gene in pituitary tumors. Cancer Res 57:5446–5451

Zhuang Z, Vortmeyer AO, Pack S, Huang S, Pham TA, Wang C, Park WS, Agarwal SK, Debelenko LV, Kester MB, Guru SC, Manickam P, Olufemi SE, Yu F, Heppner C, Crabtree JS, Skarulis MC, Venzon DJ, , Emmert-Buck MR, Spiegel AM, Chandrasekharappa SC, Collins FS, Burns AL, Marx SJ, Jensen RT, Liotta LA, Lubensky IA (1997b) Somatic mutations of the MEN1 tumor suppressor gene in sporadic gastrinomas and insulinomas. Cancer Res 57:4682–4686

Zimmer T, Ziegler K, Bäder M, Fett U, Hamm B, Riecken EO, Wiedenmann B (1994) Localisation of neuroendocrine tumours of the upper gastrointestinal tract. Gut 35:471–475

Zimmer T, Stölzel U, Bäder M, Fett U, Foss HD, Riecken EO, Rehfeld JF, Wiedenmann B (1995) A duodenal gastrinoma in a patient with diarrhea and normal serum gastrin concentrations. N Engl J Med 333:334–336

The Role of LH-RH Analogues in the Adjuvant and Palliative Treatment of Breast Cancer

K. Höffken and R. Kath

Klinik und Poliklinik für Innere Medizin II (Onkologie, Hämatologie, Endokrinologie, Stoffwechselerkrankungen), Friedrich-Schiller-Universität Jena, 00740 Jena, Germany

Abstract

Ovarian ablation has a long-standing history in the treatment of metastatic breast cancer. At the end of the past century, several reports appeared on the beneficial effect of surgical removal of the ovaries in premenopausal women with advanced breast cancer. Subsequently, this treatment became the standard systemic hormone therapy for such patients. However, the disadvantage is that only a minority of patients respond, and the remainder suffer unnecessary treatment morbidity. In a random premenopausal patient population, oophorectomy produced an average 33% objective response rate. In the search for alternatives, analogues of luteinizing hormone-releasing hormone (LH-RH) have been thoroughly investigated in pre- and postmenopausal women. The results obtained have established a place for LH-RH agonists in the treatment of premenopausal women with metastatic breast cancer. In addition, these substances have replaced oophorectomy where indicated in the adjuvant hormonal treatment of premenopausal breast cancer.

Introduction

Since its introduction, hormone receptor determination has assisted in the prediction of hormone therapy effectiveness. At the end of the past century, Schinzinger (1889) and Beatson (1896) independently reported on the beneficial effect of surgical removal of the ovaries in premenopausal women with advanced breast cancer. In the decades that followed, this became the standard systemic hormone therapy for such patients, and it has resulted in nearly 70% response rates in patients with hormone receptor-positive tumors. However, a portion of patients remain who are oophorectomized unnecessarily (about one third), and there are patients with receptor-negative tumors who

Recent Results in Cancer Research, Vol. 153
© Springer-Verlag Berlin · Heidelberg 2000

might respond to hormone ablation therapy (about one tenth). In a random premenopausal patient population, oophorectomy produced an average 33% objective response rate (Henderson and Canellos 1980). For these reasons, less invasive methods of attaining a response to hormone treatment in advanced breast cancer have been sought. Initially, this was attempted by treating premenopausal patients with high doses of an antiestrogen. Results of this approach, however, are still controversial both in terms of response rates and with regard to whether it is a reliable tool for predicting the effectiveness of subsequent ovarian ablation therapy (Hoogstraten et al. 1984; Ingle et al. 1986; Pritchard et al. 1980).

During the past two decades, analogues of luteinizing hormone-releasing hormone (LH-RH) have been thoroughly investigated in pre- and postmenopausal women (Harvey et al. 1981, 1984; Klijn and de Jong 1982, 1985; Waxman et al. 1985; Williams et al. 1986). Soon after the introduction of LH-RH agonists designed for the treatment of primary sterility or endometriosis, it became apparent that these substances induced a down-regulation of pituitary receptors, thus leading to a sustained hypogonadotropic ovarian insufficiency. Subsequent preclinical studies showed LH-RH agonists to be effective in a variety of hormone-dependent tumors, including DMBA-induced mammary tumors in female rats (Nicholson and Maynard 1979; Schally et al. 1984).

Structure, Pharmacology and Endocrinology

The development of analogues of gonadotropin (luteotropic hormone)-releasing hormone (also termed GnRH) represents an important pharmaceutical contribution. LH-RH analogues are synthetic derivatives of the natural decapeptide (Fig. 1), obtained by chemical substitution of amino acids in positions 6 and 10. The different analogues, their amino acid substitution and routes of administration are listed in Table 1. These substances show increased biological activity due to higher binding affinity and reduced degradation. When administered chronically they show sustained suppression of gonadotropin and, consequently, of sexual steroid secretion. Prior to this down-regulation at the pituitary level, an initial stimulation of gonadotropins and ovarian sexual steroids is elicited. This is the reason for naming these compounds agonists, or superagonists, of the natural LH-RH. Eventually, the result is the endocrine constellation of hypogonadotropic hypogonadism, or "medical castration". On this basis, LH-RH

1	2	3	4	5	6	7	8	9	10
pGlu	- His	- Trp	- Ser	- Tyr	- Gly	- Leu	- Arg	- Pro	- Gly-NH$_2$

Fig. 1. Amino acid sequence of the natural gonadotropin-releasing hormone agonist (LH-RH)

Table 1. Name, amino acid substitutions, and routes of administration of selected gonadotropin-releasing hormone agonists (*i.m.* intramuscular, *i.n.* intranasal, *s.c.* subcutaneous)

Name	Substitution		Routes
	Position 6	Position 10	
Leuprorelin	D-Leu	NEt	s.c., depot (i.m. or s.c.)
Triptorelin	D-Trp		s.c., depot (i.m. or s.c.)
Buserelin	D-Ser(tBu)	NEt	i.n., s.c., depot (i.m. or s.c.)
Goserelin	D-Ser(tBu)	aza-Gly	Depot (s.c.)

agonists have been successfully introduced into the treatment of hormone-dependent tumors.

Experimental Studies

Table 2 (Savino et al. 1992) outlines the development and experimental mainstays of LH-RH agonists for their use in hormone treatment of breast cancer. Important findings include the in vivo growth inhibition of tumor cell lines and experimental animal tumors and the demonstration of specific receptors for LH-RH on tumor cells.

Premenopausal Patients

Preoperative (Neoadjuvant) Treatment with LH-RH Agonists

Following the demonstration of clinical efficacy of LH-RH agonists in metastatic breast cancer, studies have been undertaken to prove the clinical benefit of this treatment on primary breast cancer sensitive to hormone therapy. Table 3 summarizes the study by Gazet et al. (1996), showing that treatment of premenopausal breast cancer patients with leuprolide resulted in 54% complete or partial remissions of the primary breast tumor. This clinical effect compares with a 60% remission rate of primary breast cancer treated with chemotherapy (mitomycin, mitoxantrone, methotrexate) or 80% with taxoid-contain-

Table 2. Summary of experimental data on LH-RH effects on breast cancer

Reference	Subject
DeSombre et al. (1976)	In vivo tumor growth inhibition of hormone-dependent neoplasia in rats
Eidne et al. (1985)	LH-RH receptors in a human breast cancer cell line (UCT Brl)
Miller et al. (1985)	Human breast cancer cell line (MCF-7) growth inhibition
Eidne et al. (1987)	Cell proliferation inhibition is not due to a protein synthesis blockage and is thus not related to a toxic effect
Scambia et al. (1988)	Inhibition of tumor growth is influenced by estrogens but does not occur through a hormone-receptor-mediated mechanism. LH-RH-A inhibit insulin and EGF-activated cell proliferation
Sharoni et al. (1989)	Inhibition of cell proliferation occurs through interference with membrane mechanisms responsible for cell activation

Table 3. Clinical assessment at 12 weeks of 13 premenopausal patients with breast cancer receiving leuprolide treatment (modified according to Gazet et al. 1996)

Response	T-stage	
	T1/2 (n)	T3/4 (n)
Complete response	2	0
Partial remission	4	1
No change	1	3
Progressive disease	2	0

ing regimens. Both treatment modalities were superior to the 35% remission rate in postmenopausal patients treated with the aromatase inhibitor formestane. Thus, LH-RH agonists warrant further investigation in preoperative breast cancer treatment.

Adjuvant Treatment with LH-RH Agonists

There is evidence that gonadal suppression is effective in reducing the risk of recurrent disease. This has been shown by studies on the correlation between chemotherapy-induced amenorrhea and relapse-free survival, by the better survival of patients treated with adjuvant chemotherapy in conjunction with oophorectomy, and by a meta-analysis of the effect of adjuvant oophorectomy on relapse-free survival or overall survival in premenopausal patients with primary breast cancer.

Existing data from studies comparing adjuvant oophorectomy or LH-RH agonist treatment with adjuvant chemotherapy suggests that there is little or no difference between the two in relapse-free survival in distinct patient subgroups, e.g., those with receptor-positive tumors. However, the data from a large phase-III trial comparing goserelin with cyclophosphamide, methotrexate, and 5-fluorouracil (CMF) as adjuvant therapy in the management of node-positive stage-II breast cancer in pre-/perimenopausal women aged 50 years or less are not yet fully available (Jonat et al. 1998). Another study (CROCTA 2) was performed in 244 pre-/perimenopausal patients with breast cancer comparing 5 years of tamoxifen treatment (plus 2 years of goserelin) with six CMF cycles in the adjuvant setting. No difference has emerged so far between the two arms at a median follow-up of 62 months (Boccardo et al. 1998).

Treatment with LH-RH Agonists in Metastatic Disease

It is now generally accepted that LH-RH agonists are effective in inducing complete and partial remissions in premenopausal patients with metastatic breast cancer. After the first clinical report by Klijn and de Jong appeared in 1982, a number of investigators showed that LH-RH agonists are capable of inducing objective remissions in about 40% of premenopausal women with advanced breast cancer. These remissions lasted between 3 and more than 37 months (median, 13 months) and were not dependent on age, tumor grade, or estrogen receptor status. In a recent open, prospective, multicenter phase-III clinical trial 73 pre-/perimenopausal patients with newly diagnosed metastatic breast cancer achieved 58% disease control (CR/PR/NC) with a median time to progression of 6 months using a monthly subcutaneous depot injection of leuprorelin acetate (Untch 1998). When LH-RH therapy (goserelin) was compared with oophorectomy in premenopausal patients with metastatic disease, failure-free and overall survival were similar in patients treated with goserelin and in those who underwent oophorectomy. However, a moderate advantage for oophorectomy was not ruled out in a multicenter randomized phase-II study (Taylor et al. 1998).

Randomized comparison between oophorectomy and LH-RH agonists remains difficult, since patients often prefer medical hormone suppression. Thus, the results available from several studies have been obtained with low patient numbers. The experimentally supported evidence from nonrandomized phase-II studies, showing that LH-RH agonists are superior to oophorectomy due to their direct cellular effect, still needs to be proven in clinical studies.

Combination of LH-RH Agonists with Other Antineoplastic Treatment Modalities

It is tempting to investigate the principle of combining several hormone preparations in order to increase efficacy and duration of remission. No convincing results have been obtained by combining traditional compounds (e.g., antiestrogens, progestins) for the treatment of hormone-sensitive breast cancer. This was especially true for overall survival.

However, there are now several studies of medical gonadal ablation showing significantly higher remission rates and longer durations (time to tumor progression) when the combination of an LH-RH agonist and tamoxifen was compared randomly with LH-RH treatment or tamoxifen alone. This finding should be taken into account in future studies on adjuvant LH-RH agonist treatment.

For metastatic disease as well, the combination of LH-RH agonists and tamoxifen proved to be superior to LH-RH agonists alone in premenopausal women with advanced breast cancer (Boccardo et al. 1999). Combinations of LH-RH agonists with other hormone preparations (e.g., antiprogestins, aromatase inhibitors) or with inhibitors of growth factors have produced only circumstantial evidence for higher efficacy than that achieved with each substance on its own.

Combination of chemotherapy with hormone therapy has resulted in higher remission rates without translating into superior survival. Therefore, standard treatment guidelines include sequential hormone and cytostatic treatment for advanced breast cancer patients.

Postmenopausal Patients

For a variety of reasons, postmenopausal patients with advanced breast cancer have been treated with LH-RH agonists. There was an approximately 15% objective remission rate. Remissions lasted between 4 and more than 19 months. Thus, there is a small fraction of postmenopausal patients (GnRH-receptor positive?, perimenopausal?) who respond to LH-RH agonist treatment. However, LH-RH agonists are not recommended as the treatment of choice under these circumstances.

Prevention of Breast Cancer

Leuprolide is currently being evaluated in a pilot study of premenopausal women for the prevention of breast cancer. However, few data are available regarding the efficacy of LH-RH agonists when they are administered prior to the carcinogen in experimental animal models of carcinoma (Hollingsworth et al. 1998).

Toxicity

Premenopausal patients experience amenorrhea and tolerable hot flushes. Hypogonadotropic hypogonadism is induced within 3 weeks of treatment begin. Castration levels of estradiol and progesterone were achieved 3 weeks after initiation of buserelin. At the same time, LH decreased significantly, and FSH remained in the range of pretherapeutic values in spite of the suppression of ovarian hormones.

When treatment is terminated in patients with no clinical benefit, resumption of sexual steroid production depends mainly on the age of the patient. Patients older than 40–45 years of age and those who have received LH-RH agonist treatment for more than 6–12 months rarely resume ovarian function. In other patients, secretion of gonadotropins and sexual steroids resumes 2–3 months following cessation of LH-RH agonist administration.

Rarely, a polyarthritis (rheumatoid) syndrome may occur that resolves after treatment is stopped (a well-documented case report is now in preparation).

Discussion

LH-RH agonist treatment is effective in treating premenopausal patients with advanced breast cancer. In view of the response rates and response durations observed with ovarian ablation therapy by LH-RH agonists, it is generally acknowledged that chemical castration by these substances may replace oophorectomy. A note of caution is necessary, however, since Williams et al. (1986) observed four patients who responded to surgical castration but failed to respond to LH-RH analogue treatment. This question has obviously not yet been addressed systematically enough to allow a definite answer. Moreover, the traditional approach to treating premenopausal patients with advanced breast cancer has been to irreversibly eliminate ovarian function, so that after a transient remission other means of hormone treatment (e.g., antiestrogens, aromatase inhibitors) are faced with only minimal residual hormone activity, such as estrogens produced by the aromatization of adrenal androgens. Therefore, it remains to be shown whether or not LH-RH agonist treatment has to provide a hormonal environment for the efficacy of subsequent hormone therapy.

On the other hand, there is suggestive evidence that LH-RH agonists directly inhibit tumor cell growth (Eidne et al. 1987; Foekens et al. 1986). This is supported by reports on the efficacy of these drugs in postmenopausal women (Harvey et al. 1981; Plowman et al. 1986).

With regard to the hormonal changes induced by treatment with LH-RH agonists, the majority of patients reached castration levels after 3 weeks of therapy.

Conclusions

LH-RH agonist treatment of pre-/perimenopausal patients with advanced breast cancer is effective, with response rates and remission durations comparable to those following oophorectomy. There is some (circumstantial) evidence for the efficacy of LH-RH agonist treatment in postmenopausal patients with advanced breast cancer.

The role of LH-RH agonists in the adjuvant therapy of premenopausal patients with primary breast cancer is under study. There is highly suggestive evidence for such a role from preliminary studies and meta-analysis data.

Preoperative (neoadjuvant) treatment with LH-RH agonists, as one of a combination or alone, is still of an experimental nature. Toxicity of LH-RH agonists is limited to menopausal symptoms. Rare other side effects include rheumatoid symptoms.

References

Beatson GT (1896) On the treatment of inoperable cases of carcinoma of the mamma: suggestions for a new method of treatment with illustrative cases. Lancet 2:104–107, 162–165
Boccardo F, Rubagotti A, Amoroso D, Mesiti M, Pacini P, Gallo L, Sismondi P, Giai M, Genta F, Mustacchi G, Agostara B, Bolognesi A, Villa E, Schieppati G, Ausili-Cefaro G, Bellantone R, Farris A, Sassi M, Patrone F (1998) Italian breast cancer adjuvant chemo-hormone therapy cooperative trials. Recent Results Cancer Res 152:453–470
Boccardo F, Blamey R, Klijn J, Tominaga T, Duchatean L, Sylvester R (1999) LH-RH agonist (LH-RH) + tamoxifen (TAM) versus LH-RH-A alone in premenopausal women with advanced breast cancer (ABC): results of a meta-analysis of four trials. Proc Am Soc Clin Oncol 18:110a (abstract 416)

DeSombre E, Johnson E, White W (1996) Regression of rat mammary tumors effected by a gonadoliberin analog. Cancer Res 36:3830–3833

Eidne K, Flanagan C, Millar R (1985) Gonadotropin-releasing hormone binding sites in human breast carcinoma. Science 229:989

Eidne K, Flanagan C, Harris N, Millar R (1987) Gonadotropin-releasing hormone (GnRH)-binding sites in human breast cancer cell lines and inhibitory effects of GnRH antagonists. J Clin Endocrinol Metab 64:425–432

Foekens JA, Henkeiman M, Fukkink J, Blankenstein M, Klijn J (1986) Direct effects of LHRH analogs on tumor cells. Eur J Cancer 22:725 (Abstr. III-s)

Gazet J-C, Coombes R, Ford H, Griffin M, Corbishley C, Markinde V, Lowndes S, Quilliam J, Sutcliffe R (1996) Assessment of the effect of pretreatment with neoadjuvant therapy on primary breast cancer. Br J Cancer 73:758–762

Harvey HA, Lipton A, Santen R, Escher G, Hardy M, Glode L, Segatoff A, Landau R, Schneir H, Max D (1981) Phase II study of a gonadotropin-releasing hormone analogue (Leuprolide) in postmenopausal advanced breast cancer patients. Proc Am Assoc Cancer Res Am Soc Clin Oncol 22:444 (Abstr. C-436)

Harvey HA, Lipton A, Max D, Pearlman H, Diaz-Porches R, de la Garza J (1984) Effective medical castration produced by the GnRH analog leuprolide in metastatic breast cancer. Proc Am Soc Clin Oncol 3:111 (Abstr. C-435)

Henderson IC, Canellos G (1980) Cancer of the breast, the past decade. Part 1. N Engl J Med 302:17–30

Hollingsworth A, Lerner M, Lightfoot S, Wilkerson K, Hanas J, McCay P, Brackett D (1998) Prevention of DMBA-inducted rat mammary carcinomas comparing leuprolide, oophorectomy, and tamoxifen. Breast Cancer Res Treat 47:63–70

Hoogstraten B, Gad-ei-Mawla N, Maloney T, Fletcher W, Vaughn C, Tranum B, Athens J, Costanzi J, Foulkes M (1984) Combined modality therapy for first recurrence of breast cancer. A Southwest Oncology Group Study. Cancer 54:2248–2256

Ingle JN, Krook J, Green S, Kubista T, Everson L, Ahmann D, Chang M, Bisel H, Windschitl H, Twito D, Pfeifle D (1986) Randomized trial of bilateral oophorectomy versus tamoxifen in premenopausal women with metastatic breast cancer. J Clin Oncol 4:178–185

Jonat W, Kaufmann M, Blamey R, Sheldon T (1998) The "ZEBRA" study: "Zoladex" (goserelin) vs CMF as adjuvant therapy in the management of node positive stage II breast cancer in pre/perimenopausal women aged 50 years or less. International Congress on Breast Cancer, San Antonio, February 27 (abstract p 107), p 41

Klijn JGM, de Jong F (1982) Treatment with a luteinising hormone-releasing hormone analogue (buserelin) in premenopausal patients with metastatic breast cancer. Lancet 1:1213–1216

Klijn JGM, de Jong F, Lamberts S, Blankenstein M (1985) LHRH-agonist treatment in clinical and experimental human breast cancer. J Steroid Biochem 23:867–873

Miller W, Scott W, Morris R, Fraser H, Sharpe R (1985) Growth of human breast cancer cells inhibited by a luteinizing hormone-releasing hormone agonist. Nature 313:231–233

Nicholson RI, Maynard P (1979) Anti-tumour activity of ICI 11863 0, a new potent luteinizing hormone-releasing hormone agonist. Br J Cancer 39:268–273

Plowman P, Nicholson R, Walker K (1986) Remissions of metastatic breast cancer in postmenopausal women with luteinising hormone-releasing hormone (ICI 11863 0) therapy. Eur J Cancer 22:746 (Abstr. 111-18)

Pritchard KI, Thomson D, Myers R, Sutherland D, Mobbs B, Meakin L (1980) Tamoxifen therapy in premenopausal patients with metastatic breast cancer. Cancer Treat Rep 64:787–796

Savino L, Baldini B, Susini T, Pulli F, Antignani L, Massi G (1992) GnRH analogs in gynecological oncology: a review. J Chemother 4:312–320

Scambia G, Benedetti Panici P, Baiocchi G, Gaggini C, Iacobelli S, Manciso S (1988) Growth inhibitory effect of LH-RH analogs on human breast cancer cells. Anticancer Res 8:187–190

Schally AV, Redding T, Comaru-Schally A (1984) Potential use of analogs of luteinizing hormone-releasing hormones in the treatment of hormone-sensitive neoplasms. Cancer Treat Rep 68:281–289

Schinzinger AS (1889) Über Carcinoma mammae. Zbl Chir (Beil) 16:55–56

Sharoni Y, Bosin E, Minister A, Levy J, Schally A (1989) Inhibition of growth of human mammary tumors cells by potent antagonists of luteinizing hormone-releasing hormone. Proc Natl Acad Sci USA 86:1648–1651

Taylor C, Green S, Dalton W, Martino S, Rector D, Ingle J, Robert N, Budd G, Paradelo J, Natale R, Bearden J, Mailliard J, Osborne C (1998) Multicenter randomized clinical trial of goserelin versus surgical ovariectomy in premenopausal patients with receptor-positive metastatic breast cancer: an intergroup study. J Clin Oncol 16:994–999

Untch M (1998) Endokrine Primärtherapie des prä- bzw. perimenopausalen Mammakarzinoms mit Leuprorelinacetat-Depot. Deutsche Leuprorelin-Studiengruppe. Zbl Gynäkol 120:286–292

Waxman JH, Harland S, Coombes R, Wrigley P, Malpas J, Powles T, Lister T (1985) The treatment of postmenopausal women with advanced breast cancer with buserelin. Cancer Chemother Pharmacol 15:171–173

Williams MR, Walker K, Turkes A, Blamey R, Nicholson R (1986) The use of an LH-RH agonist (ICI 11863 0, Zoladex) in advanced premenopausal breast cancer. Br J Cancer 53:629–636

The Combination of LH-RH Analogues with Other Treatment Modalities in Prostate Cancer

J. E. Altwein

Department of Urology, Krankenhaus der Barmherzigen Brüder, Romanstrasse 93, 80639 Munich, Germany

Abstract

Androgen deprivation is the mainstay of therapy for prostate cancer. LHRH agonists are an essential part of this form of treatment and may be employed as the only endocrine manipulation, or in combination with antiandrogens, i.e., maximal androgen blockade. In patients with bone metastases, maximal androgen blockade prolongs life for 3–6 months. The patient with minimal metastatic spread, however, may benefit much longer from this combination. In addition to being used permanently, maximal androgen blockade may be given intermittently. In locally advanced prostate cancer, LH-RH analogues, alone or together with antiandrogens, are presently being studied in conjunction with radical surgery or definitive irradiation. Whether such a neoadjuvant or adjuvant use postpones the time to progression has not yet been decided. The patient with lymph node metastases seems to benefit from early androgen deprivation in conjunction with radical prostatectomy, if the primary tumor is diploid.

Introduction

The prostate-specific antigen (PSA)-driven increase in American Joint Committee for Cancer (AJCC) stage II (comparable to $T_2N_{x,0}$ or $_1M_0$) from 25.6% in 1984 to 48.6% in 1993 and a decline in stage IV from 27.3% to 11.6% are paralleled by a decline in androgen deprivation as initial treatment (Fig. 1; Mettlin 1997) from 49.4% in 1974 to 11.0% in 1993. This trend, however, is not universally observed. The Tumor Registry of Munich reported the following figures: TNM stage II ($T_2N_0M_0$) 25.9%, stage III ($T_3N_0M_0$) 40.4%, N_+ 3.7% and M_1 11.2% (Hölzel et al. 1996). The discrepancy is even greater if the figures for initial hormone therapy are given: 38.1% of patients received androgen deprivation as the only treatment, and an additional 20.5% had

Recent Results in Cancer Research, Vol. 153
© Springer-Verlag Berlin · Heidelberg 2000

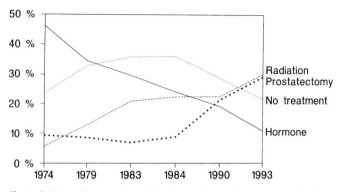

Fig. 1. Evolution of treatment modalities for carcinoma of the prostate (Mettlin 1997)

Table 1. Distribution of hormone therapy (in percent) by tumor grade, stage, and age (from Mettlin et al. 1997)

	Percent/total number of patients treated
Grade	
1	5.3/46,328
2	8.6/129,386
3	21.7/48,178
4	24.9/2291
Unknown	17.8/25,233
Stage	
0	2.6/8848
I	6.6/48,318
II	5.6/102,378
III	6.2/33,387
IV	48.6/25,954
Unknown	16.5/32,531
Age (years)	
50–64	6.4
65–69	7.6
70–74	10
75+	21

an adjuvant endocrine treatment, following either radiotherapy or radical prostatectomy. Thus, androgen deprivation may still be called the mainstay of therapeutic options employed in prostate cancer (Table 1).

Action of Androgen Deprivation

Androgen deprivation is generally considered a palliative form of treatment. This is particularly the case if the carcinoma of the prostate has a high degree of differentiation, such as Gleason score 5–7 or even 8–10. However, it ought to be mentioned that the survival of patients with a local or regional carcinoma of the prostate and Gleason score 2–4 who are an average of 71 years old and are treated with androgen deprivation is comparable to that of a group of normal men not suffering from prostate cancer (Albertsen et al. 1995).

The length of time until patients with symptomatic tumors experience relief varies with the form of androgen deprivation, partial or maximal. An example is the randomized trial of Béland (1991): Patients treated with orchiectomy plus nilutamide became free of bone pain during a follow-up of 6 months to a significantly larger extent in comparison to patients treated with orchiectomy plus placebo. If patients suffer from bone pain at inception, LH-RH analogues alone may enhance the pain (flare phenomenon); it is thus advisable to combine the chemical castration with a pure antiandrogen (flutamide, bicalutamide, or nilutamide) or cyproterone acetate (Altwein and Faul 1990).

There are anecdotal reports of long-term survival among men with bone metastases; however, their symptom status at the time of initial treatment is unknown. In general, the time to progression after the onset of osseous metastases ranges from 18 to 24 months, and the survival time is between 30 and 36 months (Schröder 1997). This palliative action of endocrine manipulation in metastatic disease is enhanced if the form of androgen deprivation has a low side-effect profile; estrogens, for instance, did not meet this requirement.

There are a number of studies available indicating that with either low-stage primary cancers or low-volume metastases androgen deprivation delays the time to progression. Thus it possibly improves the patient's quality of life, but this rarely translates into prolonged survival. Some examples are given below.

In the second VACURG trial patients with a stage C prostate cancer were randomized to be treated with placebo or 0.2 mg, 1 mg, or 5 mg DES/day. Patients receiving 1 or 5 mg DES showed a significant delay of progression to a stage D cancer (Byar 1973).

In the Intergroup Study 0036 a subset analysis of patients with a "good prognosis" experienced a longer time to objective progression, which led as well to a prolonged overall median survival (61 and 42 months, respectively; McLeod et al. 1997). This survival benefit, however, was not found in the Intergroup Study 0105, where orchiectomy plus flutamide versus orchiectomy plus placebo were the two treatment arms (Eisenberger et al. 1997).

A third example are patients with lymph node metastases who are subjected to radical prostatectomy and endocrine manipulation. The well-known studies from the Mayo Clinic demonstrate a prolonged time to progression after radical prostatectomy with adjuvant hormone therapy (Zincke et al. 1992). Unfortunately, a prospective randomized study was never completed: an example is the NPCP trial 900. The great number of retrospective studies pretending to show a survival advantage in lymph node-positive prostate cancer after radical prostatectomy and endocrine manipulation were unable to rule out a preselection of low-volume lymph node metastases (pN_1) in the group of patients subjected to radical surgery (Kalies et al. 1997). Attempts to overcome the problems inherent to a retrospective study in creating matched pairs are inconclusive, due to small numbers (Caddedu et al. 1997).

At present, therefore, hormone therapy for prostate cancer in any stage does not qualify as curative treatment: Its action, however, may be described as preventive palliation.

Efficacy of Combined Use of LH-RH Analogues

The LH-RH analogues seem to exert their antitumor activity not only through chemical castration; they also act directly on tumor cells by blocking their LH-RH receptors (Dondi et al. 1994; Palyi et al. 1996). LH-RH agonists exert a significant and dose-dependent antiproliferative action on LNCaP and DU-145 cells, and it was confirmed that these cell lines have LH-RH receptors on the cell membranes. However, these in vitro data have not been confirmed in vivo. In patients with advanced prostate cancer, the first meta-analysis from the Prostate Cancer Trialists' Collaborative Group (1995) on maximal androgen blockade did not find a difference between medical and surgical castration. The controversy regarding the advantage of maximal androgen blockade was recently discussed (Altwein 1998). Four meta-analyses comprising over 8000 patients being treated in 33 phase-III trials demonstrate a survival advantage in metastatic prostate cancer of approximately 6 months. This survival advantage was particularly apparent when the combination of medical or surgical castration with flutamide was studied separately: At a time when 1771 of 3088 randomized patients with advanced prostate cancer were dead, the ratio of annual death rates was +9% in favor of the combination ($2\,p=0.09$). At a time when 3281 patients of 4473 initially randomized had died, the advantage was 9.4%, which was significant ($2\,p<0.01$) (Labrie 1997).

It is interesting to compare the various antiandrogens in combination with LH-RH analogues or surgical castration (Table 2). As the

Table 2. Effects of antiandrogens on annual odds of death (Labrie 1997)

Treatment	Percent reduction (SD)	
	1995	1997
A: Nilutamide	6 (7)	11 (6)
B: Flutamide	9 (5)	9 (4)
C: Cyproterone acetate	−2 (11)	−9 (7)
A+B (+C)	6.4	9.4

Table 3. Best studies on maximal androgen deprivation

Study	Anti-A	No. of patients	Response duration (months Δ)	Overall survival (months Δ)	PCA survival (months Δ)
NCI-0036	Flutamide	602	3.1	7.3	
Crawford et al.	1989		$p < 0.05$	$p < 0.05$	
McLeod et al.	1997		2.6 $p < 0.05$	7.3 $p > 0.05$	
Canadian	Nilandron	194		5.4	
Béland et al.	1991			$p < 0.05$	
EORTC 30853	Flutamide		11.1	7.3	15.1
Denis et al.	1993	327	$p = 0.008$	$p = 0.02$	$p = 0.007$
Denis et al.	1998	327	7 $p = 0.009$	7 $p = 0.04$	13 $p = 0.008$
	Nilandron	423	4.1	4.1	7.3 (NS)
Janknegt et al.	1993		$p = 0.006$		
Dijkman et al.	1997		6.5	4.1	7.2
			$p = 0.002$	$p = 0.03$	$p = 0.01$

meta-analyses suffer from certain flaws, such as power of publication bias, heterogeneity, and an admixture of stages being included, one should take the best studies from the 33 trials. There, the survival advantage is quite acceptable (Table 3). It is of note that three of the four studies have been updated; the Intergroup Study 0036, for instance, was updated at a time when approximately 85% of the patients were dead.

The Intergroup Study 0105 is the largest single trial comparing maximum androgen deprivation versus monotherapy in metastatic carcinoma of the prostate (Table 4). It is interesting to witness that the combination of surgical castration plus flutamide was statistically more efficient in normalizing PSA (Table 4). Furthermore, it should be noted that it took 502 and 683 days from diagnosis to randomization with placebo and flutamide, respectively. This difference remains unexplained until a formal publication of this important trial appears. If one compares the two Intergroup Studies, the progression-free survival rate is higher in study 0105 (Table 5), whereas the observed survival is higher in the patients treated with an LH-RH analogue plus

Table 4. Intergroup study 0105; $n = 1387$ patients, power = 90% (Eisenberger et al. 1997)

	Orchiectomy+placebo	Orchiectomy+flutamide
All patients		
Observed survival	30	33 ($p = 0.067$)
Progression-free survival	19	20
Minimal disease		
Observed survival	51	52
Progression-free survival	46	48
PSA normalization (%)	62	74
	$p = 0.0002$	
Days from diagnosis to randomization	502	683

Table 5. Comparison of Intergroup studies 0036 and 0105: minimal disease

Year	Progression-free survival (%)		Observed survival (%)	
	Placebo	Flutamide	Placebo	Flutamide
1989 (LH-RH)	19.1 ↓	48.0	42.0 ↓	61.0 ↑
1997 (orchiectomy)	46.0 ↓	48.0	51.0 ↓	52.0 ↑

flutamide. These observations should be kept in mind when these two trials are interpreted.

Indications for Combined Use of LH-RH Analogues

Palliative Indication

At the present time, the data justify combining medical castration with pure antiandrogens in patients with painful bone metastases. Patients with lymph node or bone metastases and high co-morbidity probably will not benefit form maximal androgen blockade. Patients in excellent condition despite metastases from carcinoma of the prostate should be informed about the fact that, based on all available studies combining flutamide or nilutamide with medical castration, there is an average gain of 6 months of life compared to medical castration or surgical castration alone. Moreover, there is evidence that the time to progression is longer with a combined use of LH-RH analogues. Among the various pure antiandrogens, bicalutamide is probably tolerated best. The combination of cyproterone acetate with an LH-RH agonist is not better than either compound alone. Patients with minimal disease, such as solitary bone metastases confined to the axial skeleton, may benefit from longer time to progression and longer survival. This supposition is based on the Intergroup 0036 and the EORTC 30853 trials. The combination of flutamide with surgical castration is apparently not better than orchiectomy plus placebo in treating patients with minimal disease.

The following observations deserve further study. The rate of PSA normalization is higher when the combination of orchiectomy plus flutamide is used (Eisenberger et al. 1997). However, it remains to be seen whether this holds true for the combination of an LH-RH agonist with a pure antiandrogen. Quality of life was measured just recently, and the emerging data demonstrate an improvement of quality of life in patients treated with the maximal androgen blockade (Shpall 1997).

The antiandrogen withdrawal syndrome may be used as an argument for the maximal androgen blockade, as it may persist for up to 12 months after withdrawal of the antiandrogen (Collinson and Tyrrell 1994).

Neoadjuvant Use

The value of neoadjuvant hormone treatment prior to radical prostatectomy is debatable and was recently summarized (Schulman et al. 1997): Most authors have demonstrated down-sizing of the prostate in 30–50%. A clinical down-staging was demonstrated in about 30%, and there is a reduction in surgical resection margins up to 25%, although the latter has to be tested using monoclonal antibodies against specific cytokeratins and/or PSA. There are at least four prospective, randomized trials underway; intermediate results show that a prolonged survival is not very likely. Most authors have used partial androgen blockade to achieve the neoadjuvant treatment effect. Two groups, however, relied on combining an LH-RH agonist with flutamide (Labrie et al. 1994; Bellavance and Fradet 1996). They reported better responses as far as negativity of surgical margins is concerned, using such a combination preoperatively.

Similarly, neoadjuvant hormone therapy was used before radiotherapy. Again some authors propose maximal androgen blockade. So far, the ongoing phase-III trials do not permit definite conclusions. The rate of positive biopsies may be significantly reduced. However, the same arguments may be valid as in the assumption that neoadjuvant hormone treatment before radical prostatectomy lowers the positive surgical margin rate. Special staining techniques of the biopsy course are required to give a definite answer. An extensive survey of this issue was recently published (Roach 1997). At any rate, two major prospective, randomized trials have demonstrated an improvement in disease-free survival and local control using neoadjuvant combined with androgen blockade. In the protocol RTOG 8610 particularly, patients with T_{2b}–T_4 prostate cancers were randomized to receive either radiation therapy alone or LH-RH agonist plus flutamide 2 months prior to and during radiotherapy. An improvement in local control and time to PSA failure was achieved. So far, this does not translate into a prolonged survival (Pilepich et al. 1995).

Adjuvant Hormone Therapy

Patients at risk of local or systemic failure following radical prostatectomy have positive margins, seminal vesicle invasion, or high-grade (Gleason score 8–10) cancer. For these patients, a summary of the scant data may be interpreted as showing that early hormone therapy is better than late therapy (Andriole 1997). At present, however, delaying the time to progression does not translate into a longer survival. Maximal androgen blockade as adjuvant treatment for patients at high risk of local or systemic failure following radical prostatectomy has not been properly tested. The drawback might be that in these potentially long-living patients maximal androgen blockade may pose a heavy burden due to side effects. A better option would be intermittent androgen deprivation in combination with LH-RH agonists. A study under the auspices of the *Arbeitsgemeinschaft Urologische Onkologie der Deutschen Krebsgesellschaft* is under way.

Intermittent Combined Androgen Blockade

This concept is presently being studied in phase-III trials in metastatic prostate cancer. The therapeutic concept is to increase the quality of life and survival of men with advanced prostate cancer while decreasing the cost of therapy. Akakura et al. (1993) demonstrated that in the androgen-dependent Shionogi mammary cancer model, cyclic androgen withdrawal results in delayed development of androgen independence. This is felt to be related to the maintenance of the apoptotic potential. The largest trial so far conducted under the supervision of the EORTC recruited 520 patients. Reliable data are not yet available.

Summary and Conclusion

Androgen deprivation is rarely given with curative intent. If a combined androgen blockade is given to patients with metastases, time to progression and survival are prolonged. Higher costs and side effects have to be taken into account. The patient with metastases has to be informed about what to expect from combining LH-RH analogues with pure antiandrogens. The combination with cyproterone acetate does not appear to be useful.

Intermittent combined androgen blockade is presently being tested in four international prospective trials of patients with metastases. No interim data are available as yet. Thus intermittent androgen deprivation remains an experimental therapeutic concept.

Neoadjuvant or adjuvant combined androgen deprivation has been used by some authors in combination with radical prostatectomy or irradiation. There are some benefits to using certain surrogate parameters: positive margins, positive biopsies, symptom control, and local failure. However, there is currently no evidence that this leads to a prolonged survival period.

References

Akakura K, Bruchovsky N, Goldenberg SL, Rennie PS, Buckley AR, Sullivan LD (1993)) Effects of intermittent androgen suppression of androgen dependent tumors. Apoptosis and serum prostatic specific antigen. Cancer 71:2782

Albertsen PC, Fryback DG, Storer BE (1995) Long-term survival among men with conservatively treated localized prostate cancer. JAMA 274:626–631

Altwein JE (1998) Komplette Androgenblockade versus Monotherapie. Urologe A 37:149–152

Altwein JE, Faul P (1990) Probleme und Prinzipien des fortgeschrittenen Prostatakarzinoms. Klin Wochenschr 68:347–358

Andriole GL (1997) Adjuvant therapy for prostate cancer patients at high risk of recurrence following radical prostatectomy. Eur Urol 32 [Suppl 3]:65–69

Béland G (1991) Combination of anandron with orchiectomy in treatment of metastatic prostate cancer: results of a double-blind study. Urology 37 [Suppl 2]:25–29

Bellavance G, Fradet Y (1996) Influence of neoadjuvant hormonotherapy on PSA response and pathological stage at radical prostatectomy (abstract). J Urol 155 [Suppl]:1360

Byar DP (1973) The Veterans Administration Cooperative Urological Research Group's studies of cancer of the prostate. Cancer 32:1126–1130

Caddedu JA, Partin AW, Epstein JI, Walsh PC (1997) Stage D1 (T1–3, N1–3, M0) Prostate cancer: a case-controlled comparison of conservative treatment versus radical prostatectomy. Urology 50:251–255

Collinson MP, Tyrrell CJ (1994) Response of carcinoma of the prostate to withdrawal of flu-tamide. Br J Urol 73:601

Crawford ED, Eisenberger MA, McLeod DG, Spaulding JT, Benson R, Dorr FA, Blumenstein BA, Davis MA, Goodman PJ (1989) A controlled trial of leuprolide with and without flu-tamide in prostatic carcinoma. N Engl J Med 321:419–424

Denis LJ, Whelan P, De Moura JL, Newlings D, Bono A, De Pauw M (1993) Goserelin acetate and flutamide versus bilateral orchiectomy: a phase II EORTC trial (30853). Urology 42:119–130

Denis LJ, Keuppens F, Smith PH, Whelan P, Carneiro de Moura JL, Newling D, Bone A, Syl-vester R (1998) Maximal androgen blockade: final analysis of EORTC phase III trial 30853. Eur Urol 33:144–151

Dijkman GA, Janknegt RA, Reijke TM, Debruyne FMJ, Anandron Study Group (1997) Long-term efficacy and safety of nilutamide penis castration in advanced prostate cancer and the significance of early PSA normalization. J Urol 158:160–163

Dondi D, Limonta P, Moreti RM et al (1994) Antiproliferative effects of luteinizing hormone-releasing hormone (LHRH) agonists on human androgen-independent prostate cancer cell line DU 145: evidence for an autocrine-inhibitory LHRH loop. Cancer Res 54:4091–4095

Eisenberger M, Crawford ED, McLeod D, Loehrer P, Wilding G, Blumenstein B (1997) A comparison of bilateral orchiectomy (orch) with or without flutamide in stage D2 pros-tate cancer (PC) (NCI INT-0105 SWOG/ECOG). Proc ASCO 16:2A

Hölzel D, Klamert A, Schmidt M (1996) Krebs. Häufigkeiten, Befunde und Behandlungser-gebnisse. Zuckschwerdt, Munich, pp 361–372

Jangknegt RA, Abbou CC, Bartoletti R, et al (1993) Orchiectomy and anandron (nilutamide) or placebo as treatment of metastatic prostatic cancer in a multinational double-blind randomized trial. J Urol 149:77–83

Kalies R, Leitenberger A, Schneider W, Altwein JE (1997) Radikale Prostatektomie beim lymphknotenmetastasierten Prostatakarzinom? Aktuel Urol 28:309–317

Labrie F (1997) Debate: does total androgen blockade make a difference? Société Internatio-nale d'Urologie. 24th congress, Montreal, Sept. 7–11

Labrie F, Cusan L, Gomez JL, Diamond P, Suburu R, Leenay M, Tetu B, Fradet Y, Cansas B (1994) Downstaging of early stage prostate cancer before radical prostatectomy: the first randomized trial of neoadjuvant combination therapy with flutamide and a luteinizing hormone-releasing agonist. Urology 44:29–37

McLeod DG, Crawford ED, DeAntoni EP (1997) Combined androgen blockade: the gold standard for metastatic prostate cancer. Eur Urol 32 [Suppl 3]:70–77

Mettlin C (1997) Changes in patterns of prostate cancer care in the United States: results of American College of Surgeons Commission on Cancer Studies, 1974–1993. Prostate 32:221–226

Mettlin CJ, Menck HR, Winchester DP, Murphy GP (1997) A comparison of breast, colorec-tal, lung and prostate cancer reported to the National Cancer Data Base and the Surveil-lance, Epidemiology, and End Results program. Cancer 79:2052–2061

Palyi I, Vincze B, Kalnay A, et al (1996) Effect of gonadotropin-releasing hormone analogs and their conjugates on gonadotropin-releasing hormone receptor positive human can-cer lines. Cancer Detect Prevent 20:146–152

Pilepich MV, Krall JM, Al-Sarraf M, John MJ, Doggett RLS, Sause WT, Lawton CA, Abrams RA, Rotman M, Rubin P, Shipley WU, Grignon D, Caplan R, Cox JD (1995) Androgen depriva-tion with radiation therapy alone for locally advanced prostatic carcinoma: a randomized comparison trial of the Radiation Therapy Oncology Group. Urology 45:616–623

Prostate Cancer Trialists' Collaborative Group (1995) Maximum androgen blockade in ad-vanced prostate cancer: an overview of 22 randomised trials with 3283 deaths in 5710 patients. Lancet 346:265–269

Roach M III (1997) Neoadjuvant therapy prior to radiotherapy for clinically localized pros-tate cancer. Eur Urol 32 [Suppl 3]:48–54

Schröder FH (1997) Endocrine treatment of prostate cancer. In: Walsh PC, Retik AB, Vaugh-an ED, Wein AJ (eds) Campbell's urology, 7th edn, vol 2. Saunders, Philadelphia, pp 2627–2644

Shpall (1997) Health-related quality of life in men undergoing different treatments for advanced prostate cancer. J Urol 157:333A

Schulman CC, Wildschutz T, Zlotta AR (1997) Neoadjuvant hormonal treatment prior to radical prostatectomy: facts and open questions. Eur Urol 32 [Suppl 3]:41–47

Zincke H, Bergstrahl EJ, Larson-Keller JJ, Farrow GM, Myers RP, Lieber MM, Barrett DM, Rife CC, Gonchoroff NJ (1992) Stage D1 prostate cancer treated by radical prostatectomy and adjuvant hormonal treatment. Cancer 70:311–323

Primary and Salvage Therapy with LH-RH Analogues in Ovarian Cancer

G. Emons[1] and K.-D. Schulz[2]

[1] Georg-August-Universität Göttingen, Gynäkologie und Geburtshilfe,
Robert-Koch-Strasse 40, 37075 Göttingen, Germany

[2] Zentrum für Frauenheilkunde und Geburtshilfe, Philipps-Universität Marburg,
Pilgrimstein 3, 35037 Marburg, Germany

Abstract

The efficacy of modern surgical and chemotherapeutic options for the treatment of ovarian cancer is still unsatisfactory. In spite of the availability of new cytotoxic agents, the majority of ovarian cancer patients will finally die of chemoresistant disease. LH-RH agonists in conventional doses have been shown to induce objective responses in approximately 9% of patients with refractory ovarian cancer and disease stabilization in 26% of these women. As toxicity of LH-RH agonists is low or absent, and since their efficacy is not strikingly inferior to that of experimental chemotherapy, they have a vital indication in the salvage situation. A trial is presently being performed among platinum/taxol-refractory patients, comparing the impact of the LH-RH agonist leuprorelin and that of the cytotoxic agent treosulfane on survival and quality of life. The addition of LH-RH agonists in conventional doses to standard first-line surgical and chemotherapy does not improve relapse-free and overall survival. For many years it has been suggested that LH-RH agonists inhibit proliferation of ovarian cancer by suppressing endogenous gonadotropins, which were considered to be mitogenic in this malignancy. Recent experimental and clinical data have made this hypothesis questionable. In contrast, a large body of experimental evidence has emerged during the past few years indicating that LH-RH agonists and antagonists directly inhibit proliferation of ovarian cancer through LH-RH receptors expressed by 80% of these tumors. To exploit these direct antiproliferative effects of LH-RH analogues, higher tissue concentrations are necessary than those achieved with the conventional doses used today. Alternative routes of administration or higher systemic doses of potent LH-RH antagonists, such as Cetrorelix, might improve the efficacy of this approach. Clinical trials addressing this issue are under way. Finally, the LH-RH receptors expressed by ovarian cancers could be employed for targeted chemotherapy using cytotoxic LH-RH analogues. This

Recent Results in Cancer Research, Vol. 153
© Springer-Verlag Berlin · Heidelberg 2000

approach has been shown to be effective in experimental models and might be tested in clinical trials in the near future.

Introduction

Epithelial ovarian cancer is the most common fatal cancer of the female reproductive tract in the Western world and is a leading cause of cancer death among Northern American and European women (Banks et al. 1997). Despite efforts aimed at early detection, most cases are diagnosed at an advanced stage. Cytoreductive surgery in combination with platinum and, lately, taxane-based chemotherapy has produced substantial clinical improvement in these patients yielding high response rates (up to 80%) and increased short- and medium-term survival (Hoskins 1994; McGuire et al. 1996; Ozols 1997). Unfortunately, the majority of these patients eventually relapse and ultimately die of chemoresistant disease (Ozols 1997). Though the above strategy might increase long-term survival in some favorable subgroups (Neijt 1994), the overall effects on survival have been poor (Ozols 1997). To date, all available cytotoxic drugs, including topotecan and gemcitabine have a less than 25% response rate in drug-resistant ovarian cancer patients (Ozols 1997). Although clinically important palliation can be achieved with second-line treatment, including high-dose chemotherapy with autologous stem-cell transplantation, long-term survival does not seem to be significantly improved (Ozols 1997). Thus, in addition to the critical need to identify new drugs which are active in ovarian cancer, it is important to develop rational therapeutic strategies in the relapsed/refractory setting which focus on optimizing quality of life and prolonging the time to development of symptomatic disease, as well as on extending overall survival in this malignancy (Markman et al. 1996).

Hormone therapy of epithelial ovarian cancer has been investigated by clinical researchers over the past several decades (Emons and Schulz 1996). These trials, most involving only limited numbers of patients with advanced refractory ovarian cancer, have yielded average response rates of 9% (tamoxifen), 13% (progestagens), and 14%–17% (combination of progestagens and estrogens; Emons and Schulz 1996). In the majority of these trials a significant percentage of patients experienced relevant disease stabilization (Emons and Schulz 1996). Using androgens or antiandrogens, no objective responses were observed (Kavanagh et al. 1987; van der Vange et al. 1995). Recently, a large phase-II trial of tamoxifen in previously treated patients with epithelial ovarian cancer, performed by the Gynecologic Oncology Group, resulted in an objective response rate of 13% in patients with cisplatin-refractory disease (ten of 77 patients), while three (15%) of 20 patients who were cisplatin-sensitive responded (Markman et al. 1996). Marth et al. (1997) treated 155 patients with chemotherapy-resistant recurrent ovarian carcinoma with tamoxifen. In the 65 patients evaluable for response there were four objective responders (6%). In 77% of evaluable patients disease was stabilized (Marth et al. 1997). Used in a first-line therapy setting, the addition of tamoxifen to chemotherapy (cisplatin plus adriamycin) had no significant effect on overall or progression-free survival of patients with stage III or IV epithelial ovarian cancer (Schwartz et al. 1989).

In 1985, Parmar and colleagues (Parmar et al. 1985) reported on a patient with advanced ovarian cancer who had relapsed after surgery, chemotherapy, and radiotherapy. Treatment with the LH-RH agonist triptorelin led to a marked shrinkage of the tumor mass that lasted for 12 months. This encouraging report stimulated intensive basic and clinical research on the use of LH-RH analogues in the treatment of ovarian cancer. The original rationale for this approach was the hypothesis that the growth of ovarian cancer was dependent on gonadotropins. In this context the suppression of endogenous LH and FSH by LH-RH agonists should have beneficial effects in patients with ovarian cancer. More recently, it became apparent that most ovarian cancers express receptors for LH-RH which might mediate direct antiproliferative effects of LH-RH analogues (Emons and Schulz 1996).

Effects of Gonadotropins on the Growth of Epithelial Ovarian Cancer

A large body of epidemiological and experimental data suggests that epithelial ovarian cancer could be dependent on gonadotropin secretion. However, a number of studies indicate that this might be not the case. This literature has been extensively reviewed (Emons et al. 1992, 1996a; Foekens and Klijn 1992; Emons and Schally 1994; Emons and Schulz 1996). Recently, this hypothesis was further supported by the demonstration of the expression of messenger ribonucleic acid expression of the LH/hCG receptor gene in human ovarian carcinomas (Mandai et al. 1997). In five of six cases of ovarian cancer developing in infertile women during or after ovulation-induction therapy, LH/hCG receptors were found (Kuroda et al. 1997). Other recent reports have contested the hypothesis that pituitary gonadotropins increase the risks of ovarian cancer (Helzlsouer et al. 1995; Hankinson et al. 1995). The current epidemiological data are insufficient to implicate conclusively specific fertility medications in ovarian carcinogenesis (Emons et al. 1996b; Bristow and Karlan 1996; Banks et al. 1997). Thus, the role of gonadotropins in the development and proliferation of epithelial ovarian cancer remains to be defined.

Direct Effects of LH-RH Analogues on the Proliferation of Ovarian Cancer

In recent years, the expression of LH-RH and its receptor has been demonstrated in a number of malignant human tumors, including cancers of the breast, ovary, endometrium, and prostate. These findings suggest the presence of an autocrine regulatory system based on LH-RH. Dose-dependent antiproliferative effects of LH-RH agonists and antagonists in cell lines derived from these cancers have been observed by various investigators (Emons and Schally 1994; Imai et al. 1994, 1996a; Emons et al. 1996b, 1997; Moretti et al. 1996). Findings from several laboratories, including ours, suggest that the classical LH-RH receptor signal-transduction mechanisms, known to operate in the pituitary, are not involved in the mediation of antiproliferative effects of LH-RH analogues in cancer cells. Data obtained during the past several years instead suggest that LH-RH analogues interfere with the mitogenic signal transduction of growth-factor receptors and related oncogene products associated with tyrosine kinase activity (Fig. 1; Imai et al. 1996b; Emons 1996a, 1997; Moretti et al. 1996; Shirahige et al. 1994). Approximately 80% of ovarian cancers express receptors for LH-RH which are probably part of a local LH-RH-based regulatory system and can mediate direct antiproliferative effects of LH-RH analogues. These receptors might be used as a point of attack for the therapy of ovarian cancer (Emons et al. 1996a, 1997).

Salvage Therapy with LH-RH Analogues in Ovarian Cancer

The successful treatment of a patient with relapsed ovarian cancer by Parmar et al. (1985) using triptorelin stimulated a number of phase-II trials on the use of LH-RH agonists in patients with relapsed ovarian cancer, mostly refractory to platinum (Table 1). Average rates of 9.4% objective responses and 26% disease stabilization were obtained. The

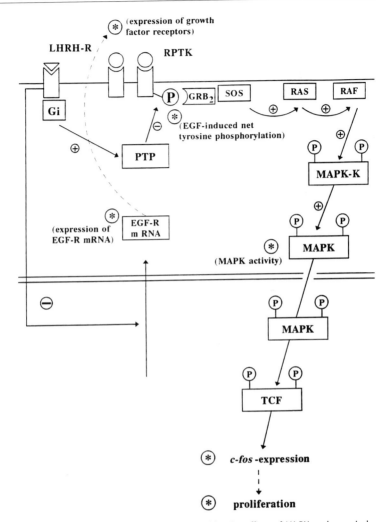

Fig. 1. Hypothetical molecular mechanisms mediating the antiproliferative effects of LH-RH analogues in human cancer cells. *Gi* Gi protein, *GRB₂* adapter protein, *LHRH-R* LH-RH receptor, *MAPK* mitogen-activated protein kinase, *MAPK-K* MAPK kinase, *PTP* phosphotyrosine phosphatase, *RAF* a protein-serine/threonine kinase, *RAS* a small GTPase of the RAS family, *RPTK* receptor protein tyrosine kinase [for example, epidermal growth factor (*EGF*) receptor], *SOS* guanine nucleotide exchange factor, *TCF* transcription factor. *Asterisk* indicates mechanisms that have been shown to be inhibited by LH-RH-analogue treatment. For references and further details see Emons et al. (1997). (From Emons et al. 1997, with permission from Elsevier Science Inc.)

duration of objective responses was 2–38+ months. Treatment toxicity was very mild or absent.

Lopez et al. (1996) recently treated 20 patients with platinum-resistant ovarian carcinoma with the LH-RH agonist leuprorelin and tamoxifen. Among the 17 evaluable patients, two women had a partial

Table 1. Results of phase-II clinical trials[a] using LH-RH agonists in relapsed, mostly platinum-resistant ovarian cancer

Reference	LH-RH agonist	Evaluable patients (n)	Complete remissions	Partial remissions	Stable disease
Parmar et al. (1988a,b)	Triptorelin	41	–	6	5
Kullander et al. (1987)	Triptorelin	10	–	2	3
Jäger et al. (1989)	Triptorelin	19	–	–	11
Bruckner and Motwani (1989)	Leuprorelin	5	1	3	1
Kavanagh et al. (1989)	Leuprorelin	18	–	4	2
Vavra et al. (1990)	Goserelin	19	–	3	5
Lind et al. (1992)	Goserelin	30	–	2	5
Miller et al. (1992)	Leuprorelin	25	–	1	15
Carmino et al. (1994)	Triptorelin	20	–	–	8
van der Vange et al. (1995)	Triptorelin	8	1	–	–
Ron et al. (1995)	Triptorelin	14	–	–	8
Jäger et al. (1995)	Triptorelin	36	–	–	1
		245	2	21	64
			9.4%		26%

[a] Duration of response 2–38+ months.

response, each lasting 7 months. Five additional patients (29%) experienced disease stabilization with a median duration of 5 months. The authors concluded that this response rate was not significantly different from those in previously published studies using either leuprorelin or tamoxifen alone. The median survival was 14.4 months, and this was not significantly different from a median survival of 11.4 months obtained by these authors in a group of patients with refractory ovarian carcinoma who received high-dose tamoxifen (Lopez et al. 1996).

In a randomized prospective trial, Jäger et al. (1995) compared the effects of the LH-RH analogue triptorelin with those of tamoxifen in 73 patients with progressive ovarian cancer in whom all established treatment modalities (e.g., repeated surgery, different chemotherapies) had failed. No clinical remission was observed in either of the two treatment groups and no differences were observed in survival. Median survival was 6 months in both groups. In the triptorelin group, LH and FSH were suppressed after initiation of treatment, while there was only a slight but not significant reduction of gonadotropin levels in the tamoxifen group. The authors concluded that the suppression of gonadotropins by the LH-RH analogue as a last-line treatment did not substantially improve the outcome in progressive ovarian cancer (Jäger et al. 1995). In our opinion, the design of this trial, using tamoxifen as a control, does not allow for this clear conclusion, as the antiestrogen has shown some activity in the salvage therapy of refractory ovarian cancer (Markman et al. 1996; Marth et al. 1997; Emons and Schulz 1996).

Only modest remission rates and disease stabilization are to be expected from LH-RH therapy in patients refractory to platinum and/or paclitaxel therapy. In this situation, however, the results of further chemotherapy are not strikingly superior (Markman et al. 1996; Ozols 1997). Given the low or absent toxicity of LH-RH analogues, they, like other endocrine agents, have a vital indication for salvage therapy, particularly when the patient's quality of life is a major concern (NIH Consensus Conference 1995).

Based on these considerations, a randomized trial is being performed in Germany. Patients with surgically treated advanced ovarian cancer who have progressive disease on platinum/paclitaxel therapy or experience an early relapse after six cycles of this treatment receive either an alkylating agent (treosulfane) or the LH-RH agonist leuprorelin. Study parameters are overall survival and toxicity (quality of life; AGO-Ovarian Cancer Group, personal communication).

Primary Therapy of Ovarian Cancer with LH-RH Analogues

Few trials have addressed the efficacy of a combination of surgery and first-line chemotherapy with LH-RH agonists in the treatment of advanced ovarian cancer. Medl et al. (1993) treated 15 patients with stage IIc–IV ovarian cancer with a combination of six courses of carboplatin-containing polychemotherapy and the LH-RH agonist triptorelin. They observed no significant differences in terms of response, survival, and time to progression compared with a historical control group. In a phase-II study by Erickson et al. (1994), 33 patients with stage III or IV ovarian cancer were surgically debulked and then treated with a combination of a cisplatin-containing polychemotherapy (six cycles) and six monthly injections of a depot preparation of leuprorelin acetate. Leuprorelin consistently suppressed FSH levels to less than 20 IU/l in all patients. However, comparisons with historical controls showed that the use of the LH-RH analogue did not alter the toxicity profile or the effectiveness of chemotherapy (Erickson et al. 1994).

We recently completed a randomized prospective multicenter trial, enrolling 135 patients with stage III or IV epithelial ovarian cancer. After cytoreductive surgery, 69 patients received monthly injections of a depot preparation of the LH-RH agonist triptorelin (3.75 mg) and

66 patients received placebo until their deaths or termination of the trial, respectively. All patients were treated with a standard platinum-based chemotherapy and, if necessary, with second- or third-line cytotoxic regimens. Endogenous gonadotropins were reliably suppressed in patients treated with triptorelin. However, their progression-free and overall survivals were not significantly different from those of patients receiving placebo injections (statistical power >80% for a difference between both groups of >20%). For us, the results of this trial suggest that the suppression of endogenous gonadotropins by conventional doses of an LH-RH agonist produces no relevant beneficial effects in patients with advanced ovarian carcinoma who receive standard surgical cytoreduction and cytotoxic chemotherapy (Emons et al. 1996c). Therefore, LH-RH agonists in conventional doses cannot be recommended in the primary therapy of ovarian cancer, except perhaps for patients who are unable or unwilling to undergo first-line chemotherapy.

Conclusions and Future Directions

The original rationale for employing LH-RH analogues in the therapy of epithelial ovarian cancer was the suppression of endogenous gonadotropins, as LH and/or FSH were considered to be mitogenic for these tumors. To date, the latter assumption is still a matter of controversy in experimental studies. The clinical trials so far performed on the basis of this rationale have been conducted using the conventional doses of LH-RH agonists, which suppress endogenous gonadotropins. In the treatment of diseases in which a suppression of gonadotropin secretion or the resulting reversible medical gonadectomy is the therapeutic aim, these conventional LH-RH agonist doses, administered mostly as slow-release preparations, have become established therapeutic options. Such diseases include idiopathic precocious puberty, endometriosis, uterine fibroids, hormone-dependent premenopausal breast cancer, and prostatic cancer (Emons and Schally 1994; Emons et al. 1996a; Schally and Comaru-Schally 1997). Also in various procedures of assisted reproduction, suppression of endogenous gonadotropins by LH-RH analogues is widely used (Emons and Schally 1994; Emons et al. 1997).

In the first-line therapy of ovarian cancer this approach probably has no substantial impact. In the salvage situation, conventional doses of LH-RH agonists seem to have marginal activity. Due to low or absent toxicity, refractoriness to platinum and taxane chemotherapies or inability or unwillingness to accept chemotherapy are vital indications for the administration of LH-RH agonists to ovarian cancer patients, particularly when quality of life is of concern.

The direct antiproliferative effects of LH-RH analogues on ovarian cancer, mediated through the LH-RH receptors present in 80% of these carcinomas, are well established in cell culture and nude mice models (Emons et al. 1997). Their clinical application, however, is just at the beginning. For the full exploitation of the direct antimitogenic effects of LH-RH analogues on cancers, significantly higher concentrations of these compounds are needed than those achieved in vivo with the conventional depot preparations of LH-RH agonists used today for the above-mentioned indications. The LH-RH agonist plasma concentrations achieved by these formulations are fully active to suppress pituitary gondotrophs but only marginally effective as regards direct antitumor effects (Emons and Schally 1994; Emons et al. 1997). Higher systemic doses of LH-RH agonists or alternative routes of administration – for instance, intraperitoneally in ovarian cancer patients – might increase the efficacy of this approach. LH-RH antagonists such as Cetrorelix have been shown to be superior to LH-RH agonists in some cancer models (Emons et al. 1996 d; Schally and Comaru-Schally 1997). A clinical trial addressing the efficacy of high doses of the LH-RH antagonist Cetrorelix in refractory ovarian cancer is under way.

The LH-RH receptors expressed by ovarian and other cancers might also be utilized for a targeted chemotherapy based on cytotoxic LH-RH analogues. This approach has been shown to be effective in several in vitro and in vivo cancer models, including human epithelial ovarian cancer (Schally et al. 1996; Jungwirth et al. 1997; Miyazaki et al. 1997). The intensive research being performed at present in this field of cytotoxic LH-RH analogues should soon lead to clinical testing and could result in more efficacious and less toxic targeted chemotherapy for the 80% of ovarian cancer patients whose malignancies express LH-RH receptors. Taking into account the present most unsatisfactory situation in the therapy of ovarian cancer, these promising novel approaches exploiting the LH-RH system expressed by these tumors deserve great attention.

References

Banks E, Beral V, Reeves G (1997) The epidemiology of epithelial ovarian cancer: a review. Int J Gynecol Cancer 7:425–438

Bristow RE, Karlan BY (1996) The risk of ovarian cancer after treatment for infertility. Curr Opin Obstet Gynecol 8:32–37

Bruckner HW, Motwani BT (1989) Treatment of advanced refractory ovarian carcinoma with a gonadotropin-releasing hormone analogue. Am J Obstet Gynecol 161:1216–1218

Carmino F, Iskra L, Fuda G, Foglia G, Odicino F, Bruzzone M, Chiara S, Gadduchi A, Ragni N for the Gruppo Oncologico Nord Ovest (GONO) (1994) The treatment of progressive ovarian carcinoma with D-Trp-LH-RH (Decapeptyl). Eur J Cancer 30A:1903–1904

Emons G, Schally AV (1994) The use of luteinizing hormone-releasing hormone agonists and antagonists in gynecological cancers. Hum Reprod 9:1364–1379

Emons G, Schulz K-D (1996) Growth regulation of epithelial ovarian cancer by hormones, peptide growth factors, and cytokines. In: Pasqualini JR, Katzenellenbogen BS (eds) Hormone-dependent cancer. Dekker, New York, pp 509–539

Emons G, Ortmann O, Pahwa GS, Oberheuser F, Schulz K-D (1992) LH-RH agonists in the treatment of ovarian cancer. In: Höffken K (ed) Peptides in oncology. I. LH-RH agonists and antagonists. Springer, Berlin Heidelberg New York, pp 55–68 (Recent results in cancer research, vol 124)

Emons G, Ortmann O, Schulz K-D (1996a) GnRH analogues in ovarian, breast and endometrial cancers. In: Lunenfeld B, Insler V (eds) GnRH analogues. The state of the art 1996. Parthenon, New York, pp 95–120

Emons G, Ortmann O, Schulz K-D (1996b) Ovulationsinduktion und Karzinomrisiko. Gynakologe 29:291–299

Emons G, Ortmann O, Teichert HM, Fassl H, Löhrs U, Kullander S, Kauppila A, Ayalon D, Schally A, Oberheuser F for the Decapeptyl Ovarian Cancer Study Group (1996c) Luteinizing hormone-releasing hormone agonist triptorelin in combination with cytotoxic chemotherapy in patients with advanced ovarian carcinoma. A prospective double-blind randomized trial. Cancer 78:1452–1460

Emons G, Ortmann O, Irmer G, Müller V, Schulz K-D, Schally AV (1996d) Treatment of ovarian cancer with LH-RH antagonists. In: Filicori M, Flamigni C (eds) Treatment with GnRH analogs: controversies and perspectives. Parthenon, New York, pp 165–172

Emons G, Ortmann O, Schulz K-D, Schally AV (1997) Growth-inhibitory actions of analogues of luteinizing hormone-releasing hormone on tumor cells. Trends Endocrinol Metab 8:355–362

Erickson LD, Hartmann LC, Su JQ, Nielsen SNJ, Pfeifel DM, Goldberg RM, Levitt R, Stanhope CR (1994) Cyclophosphamide, cisplatin and leuprolide acetate in patients with debulked stage III or IV ovarian carcinoma. Gynecol Oncol 54:196–200

Foekens JA, Klijn JGM (1992) Direct antitumor effects of LH-RH analogs. In: Höffken K (ed) Peptides in oncology. I. LH-RH agonists and antagonists. Springer, Berlin Heidelberg New York, pp 55–68 (Recent results in cancer research, vol 124)

Hankinson SE, Colditz GA, Hunter DJ, Willet WC, Stampfer MJ, Rosner B, Hennekens CH, Spreizer FE (1995) A prospective study of reproductive factors and risk of epithelial ovarian cancer. Cancer 76:284–290

Helzlsouer KJ, Alberg AJ, Gordon GB, Longcope C, Bush TL, Hoffman SC, Comstock GW (1995) Serum gonadotropins and steroid hormones and the development of ovarian cancer. J Am Med Assoc 274:1926–1930

Hoskins WJ (1994) Epithelial ovarian carcinoma: principles of primary surgery. Gynecol Oncol 55:591–596

Imai A, Ohno T, Iida K, FuseyaT, Furui T, Tamaya T (1994) Gonadotropin-releasing hormone receptors in gynecologic tumors. Cancer 74:2555–2561

Imai A, Takagi H, Furui T, Horibe S, Fuseya T, Tamaya T (1996a) Evidence for coupling of phosphotyrosine phosphatase to gonadotropin-releasing hormone receptor in ovarian carcinoma membrane. Cancer 77:132–137

Imai A, Horibe S, Takagi H, Fuseya T, Tamaya T (1996b) Signal transduction of GnRH receptor in the reproductive tract tumor. Endocr J 43:249–260

Jäger W, Wildt L, Lang N (1989) Some observations on the effects of a GnRH analog in ovarian cancer. Eur J Obstet Gynecol Reprod Biol 32:137–148

Jäger W, Sauerbrei W, Beck E, Maaßen V, Stumpfe M, Meier W, Kuhn W, Jänicke F (1995) A randomized comparison of triptorelin and tamoxifen as treatment of progressive ovarian cancer. Anticancer Res 15:2639–2642

Jungwirth A, Schally AV, Nagy A, Pinski J, Groot K, Galvan G, Szepeshaszi K, Halmos G (1997) Regression of rat dunning R-3327-H prostate carcinoma by treatment with targeted cytotoxic analog of luteinizing hormone-releasing hormone AN-207 containing 2-pyrrolinodoxorubicin. Int J Oncol 10:877–884

Kavanagh JJ, Wharton JT, Roberts WS (1987) Androgen therapy in the treatment of refractory epithelial ovarian cancer. Cancer Treat Rep 71:537–538

Kavanagh JJ, Roberts W, Townsend P, Hewitt S (1989) Leuprolide acetate in the treatment of refractory or persistent epithelial ovarian cancer. J Clin Oncol 7:115–118

Kullander S, Rausing A, Schally AV (1987) LH-RH agonist treatment in ovarian cancer. In: Klijn JGM, Paridaens R, Foekens JA (eds) Hormonal manipulation of cancer: peptides, growth factors, and new (anti)steroidal agents. Raven, New York, pp 353–356

Kuroda H, Konishi I, Mandai M, Nanbu K, Rao CV, Mori T (1997) Ovarian cancer in infertile women during or after ovulation-induction therapy: expression of LH/hCG receptors and sex steroid receptors. Int J Gynecol Cancer 7:451–457

Lind MJ, Cantwell BMJ, Millward MJ, Robinson A, Proctor M, Simmons D, Carmichael J, Harris AL (1992) A phase II trial of goserelin (Zoladex) in relapsed epithelial ovarian cancer. Br J Cancer 65:621–623

Lopez A, Tessadrelli A, Kudelka AP, Edwards CL, Freedman RS, Hord M, Kavanagh JJ (1996) Combination therapy with leuprolide acetate and tamoxifen in refractory ovarian cancer. Int J Gynecol Cancer 6:15–19

Mandai M, Konishi I, Kuroda H, Fukumoto M, Komatsu T, Yamamoto S, Nanbu K, Rao CV, Mori T (1997) Messenger ribonucleic acid expression of LH/hCG receptor gene in human ovarian carcinomas. Eur J Cancer 33:1501–1507

Markman M, Iseminger K, Hatch KD, Creasman WT, Barnes W, Dubeskter B (1996) Tamoxifen in platinum-refractory ovarian cancer: a Gynecologic Oncology Group ancillary report. Gynecol Oncol 62:4–6

Marth C, Sorheim N, Kaern J, Tropé C (1997) Tamoxifen in the treatment of recurrent ovarian carcinoma. Int J Gynecol Cancer 7:256–261

McGuire WP, Hoskins WJ, Brady MF, Kucera PR, Partridge EE, Look KY, Clarke-Pearson DL, Davidson M (1996) Cyclophosphamide and cisplatin compared with paclitaxel and cisplatin in patients with stage III and stage IV ovarian cancer. N Engl J Med 334:1–6

Medl M, Peters-Engel C, Fuchs G, Leodolter S (1993) Triptorelin (D-Trp⁶-LH-RH) in combination with carboplatin-containing polychemotherapy for advanced ovarian cancer: a pilot study. Anticancer Res 13:2373–2376

Miller DS, Brady MF, Barrett RJ (1992) A phase II trial of leuprolide acetate in patients with advanced epithelial ovarian carcinoma. Am J Clin Oncol 15:125–128

Miyazaki M, Nagy A, Schally AV, Lamharzi N, Halmos G, Szepeshazi K, Groot K, Armatis P (1997) Growth inhibition of human ovarian cancers by cytostatic analogs of luteinizing hormone releasing hormone. J Natl Cancer Inst 89:1803–1809

Moretti MR, Montagnani-Morelli M, Dondi D, Poletti A, Martini L, Motta M, Limonta D (1996) Luteinizing hormone-releasing hormone agonists interfere with the stimulatory action of epidermal growth factor in human prostatic cancer cell lines, LNCaP and DU 145. J Clin Endocrinol Metab 81:3930–3937

Neijt JP (1994) Advances in the chemotherapy of gynecologic cancer. Curr Opin Oncol 6:531–538

NIH Consensus Conference (1995) Ovarian cancer, screening, treatment, and follow-up. J Am Med Assoc 273:491–497

Ozols RF (1997) Treatment of recurrent ovarian cancer: increasing options – "recurrent" results (editorial). J Clin Oncol 15:2177–2180

Parmar H, Nicoll J, Stockdale A, Cassoni A, Phillips RH, Lightman SL, Schally AV (1985) Advanced ovarian carcinoma: response to the agonist D-Trp⁶LH-RH. Cancer Treat Rep 69:1341–1342

Parmar H, Rustin F, Lightman SL, Phillips RH, Hanham JW, Schally AV (1988a) Response to D-Trp6-luteinizing hormone-releasing hormone (decapeptyl) microcapsules in advanced ovarian cancer. Br Med J 296:1229

Parmar H, Phillips RH, Rustin F, Lightman SL, Hanham JW, Schally AV (1988b) Therapy of advanced ovarian cancer with D-Trp6-LH-RH (decapeptyl) microcapsules. Biomed Pharmacother 42:531–538

Ron IG, Wigler N, Merimsky O, Inbar MJ, Chaitchik S (1995) A phase II trial of D-Trp-6-LH-RH (decapeptyl) in pretreated patients with advanced epithelial ovarian cancer. Cancer Invest 13:272–275

Schally AV, Comaru-Schally AM (1997) Hypothalamic and other peptide hormones. In: Holland JF, Frei E III, Bast RR jr, Kufe DE, Morton DL, Weichselbaum RR (eds) Cancer medicine, 4th edn. Williams and Wilkins, Baltimore, pp 1067–1086

Schally AV, Nagy A, Szepeshazi K, Pinski J, Halmos G, Armatis P, Miyazaki M, Comaru-Schally AM, Yano T, Emons G (1996) LH-RH analogs and cytotoxic radicals. In: Filicori M, Flamigni C (eds) Treatment with GnRH analogs: controversies and perspectives. Parthenon, New York, pp 165–172

Schwartz PE, Chambers JT, Kohorn EJ, Chambers SK, Weitzman H, Voynick JM, MacLusky N, Naftolin F (1989) Tamoxifen in combination with cytotoxic chemotherapy in advanced epithelial ovarian cancer. Cancer 63:1074–1078

Shirahige Y, Cook C, Pinski J, Halmos G, Nair R, Schally AV (1994) Treatment with luteinizing hormone-releasing hormone antagonist SB-75 decreases levels of epidermal growth factor receptor and its mRNA in OV-1063 human epithelial ovarian cancer xenografts in nude mice. Int J Oncol 5:1031–1035

Van der Vange N, Greggi S, Burger CW, Kenemans P, Vermorken JB (1995) Experience with hormonal therapy in advanced epithelial ovarian cancer. Acta Oncol 34:813–820

Vavra N, Barrada M, Fitz R, Sevelda P, Bauer M, Dittrich C (1990) Goserelin – eine neue Form der Hormontherapie beim Ovarialkarzinom. Gynakol Rundsch 30 [Suppl 1]:61–63

Subject Index

Printing (Computer to Film): Saladruck, Berlin
Binding: Stürtz AG, Würzburg